DRUG DISCOVERY
The Pending Crisis

DRUG DISCOVERY
THE PENDING CRISIS
Stephen L. DeFelice, MD

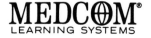

MEDC⊕M®
LEARNING SYSTEMS

Medcom Production Staff

ROBERT E. FUISZ, MD
Publisher

RICHARD C. FUISZ, MD
Publisher

DAVID P. LAULER, MD
Editor-in-Chief

VIRGINIA MALFITAN, MD
Medical Director

ROBERT B. WILSON
Executive Editor

RUTH A. ROSENBLUM
Managing Editor

ALFRED R. KELMAN
Executive Film Producer

GARY N. OLIVO
Executive Art Director

MEDICAL CONSULTANTS
Myra Freilich Boritz, MD
Stephen Moss, DDS
Peter Philander, MD
Nita Taskier, PhD

PROJECT EDITORIAL DIRECTOR
Janet Wagner

MEDICAL EDITORS
Pia Bortnowski
Claire Hillard
Sandra Pelus
Susan Rockwell
Madeleine Steele

PRODUCTION MANAGER
Joan Milarsky

ART DIRECTOR
Barbara Asch

GRAPHIC ILLUSTRATOR
Etta Siegel

MANAGER PHOTOGRAPHY AND PERMISSIONS
Helena Frost

PHOTO RESEARCH
Cathie Furbush

TECHNICAL RESEARCH
Deborah Graham

COPY STAFF
Mariam Cohen
Marion Lazos
Mary Bozeman Raines
Selma Ramsey
Elena Rosti
Susan Rubin

EDITORIAL COORDINATOR
Rose Ann Borreca

Medcom Press is a division of MEDCOM, Inc.
MEDCOM®
LEARNING SYSTEMS
World leader in multimedia health education programs
2 Hammarskjöld Plaza, New York, N. Y. 10017/(212) 832-1400

Library of Congress Catalog Number 72–87152

Printed in U.S.A.

To Stefano, Anna and Marianne Patrice

Contents

Acknowledgments

To Gerald Laubach whose knowledge of clinical drug development is unsurpassed.

To Joseph DiPalma, Leo Hollister, and Louis Lasagna, whose critiques were invaluable.

And to Shelly Gilgore for the privilege of being his associate.

Preface

The impact of the thalidomide episode on American drug development has been substantial. Not only was it responsible for the passage of the 1962 Kefauver-Harris amendments, but it lead to an ever-increasing stress on the safety of the FDA drug approval process. As a result, the loss to the public from delays in approval of important new drugs has been deemphasized, so that the U.S. now lags behind many other countries in regard to the availability of new chemical entities. (We were the 41st country to approve lithium as a psychopharmacologic agent, and the 51st country to approve the important antitubercular drug rifampin.)

In this book, Dr. DeFelice deals with the key issues in clinical drug development—the process itself and the individuals who participate in that process. If the mechanisms are faulty, inefficient, or ponderous, the public will suffer. If the men and women who are the active participants in the process are deficient in ability or training or logic, again, the sick patient pays the price. This book's important message—to me at least—is that we are stressing the nonclinical aspects of drug development too much and not stressing sufficiently the early and adequate study of drug candidates in man. These errors are in large part attributable to the noble goal, unfortunately not achieved by such emphasis, of preventing harm to the public. One cannot argue with safety measures that work; one *can* argue with those that do not, but merely provide, at great cost, the illusion of safeguards and wisdom.

LOUIS LASAGNA, MD
ROCHESTER, NEW YORK
NOVEMBER 9, 1971

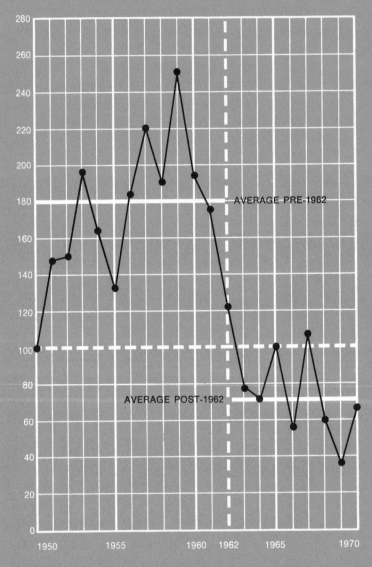

Figure 1 / New single chemical-entity introductions since 1950. (From P de Haen, *Nonproprietary Name Index*, New York, Paul de Haen, Inc, 1971. Redrawn from illustration by JP Curran.)

To Begin With

Consumerism and science are with us.

The very term consumerism signifies a basic goal of assuring the greatest good for the ultimate consumer. In the medical area of scientific research, this naturally demands the application of all reasonable safety measures to guard the public from actual or potential hazards in the usage of drugs.

But it also requires—though in far more subtle fashion—consumer protection by stimulating development of new and better drugs that lessen or eliminate disease morbidity and mortality.

The latter requirement, it seems to me, is clearly designed to benefit the consumer, and so it should be weighed relative to the consumer's interest in terms of safety. Though oftentimes very difficult to achieve, both are necessary to a degree that precludes the elimination of either one. This weighing is perhaps most comparable to two horses pulling in double harness. If one is allowed to feed at the other's expense, the second horse weakens . . . the cart founders.

Unfortunately this very situation can easily occur in medical research, and in reality, the long-range consumer benefit can be submerged by the high valuation placed upon the safety factor.

There is substantial evidence of a decline in discovery and development of new types of medicinal drugs (see Fig. 1). Perhaps even more disturbing than the actual decline, however, is the complacency with which it is being met.

Resolving this conflict of "consumerism against itself" is pro-

1

genitor to a relatively new medical specialty—*clinical drug development*—which requires broad background and training and an unusual combination of skills.

The specialist in this area—a *clinical drug developer* (CDD) —is needed right now to cope with the complex technology and regulatory standards required in drug development and clinical research, and he will be needed increasingly in the years ahead to bring more drugs to man for evaluation and to develop those valuable in the treatment of patients.

To a significant extent, the current emphasis upon consumer safety becomes understandable if one turns back the pages of history. The thalidomide tragedy in the early 1960s caused reverberations that were heard almost immediately in every household in the country. A resulting societal fear arose, and it naturally followed that there was a great demand for increased consumer protection. Also, consumerism has occurred in other areas where there were no thalidomide tragedies.

There is something larger going on in society that permits an overreaction to bad events.

Be that as it may, it has become increasingly obvious that the measures currently employed to achieve the short-range goal of guarding consumer safety have been detrimental to the long-range goal of better consumer protection through better medications. Our attempt to guard against another thalidomide episode has spawned an overemphasis on actual or potential drug toxicity; in turn, this has resulted in unhealthy restrictions on clinical research. Thus, we find today that an isolated type of animal toxicity all too often can prevent a new drug from being evaluated in man.

The rationale is clear: If toxicity occurs in animals, it may occur in man and outweigh the good achieved by the desired clinical effect. However, this often is not the case. With present methodology, the ability to draw correlations between toxic effects in animals and possible toxicity in man is far from being 100%. Similarly we have little scientific reason to believe that a drug with outstanding activity in animals will necessarily exhibit parallel clinical activity in man. After all, the life spans of animal and man vary widely; their metabolic rates may be qualitatively and quantitatively different; their variances in physiology and anatomy lead to disparate rates of absorption, biotransformation, and excretion. Indeed, when one considers the dis-

2

similarities in drug responses just between men and women or between people of African, Mediterranean, and Northern European background, one may wonder why the findings from animal screens offer even such limited correlations with man as have been found to exist! And one may rightfully wonder, too, what human diseases are still uncontrolled because the drug that would have safely cured them was too toxic, or ineffective, in dogs or rats.

Only by increasing our clinical research can we properly evaluate our existing animal screens and determine where and how they may be applied to make their use a rational and scientific one. And only in this way can we save from the laboratory morgue many potentially valuable drugs to treat major diseases.

Even a cursory examination of many important drugs on which today's physicians rely, such as the phenothiazines, discloses that many of them were discovered in man largely as a result of fortuitous circumstances. Today, however, while serendipity will probably continue to play a role in new-drug discovery, our philosophy is structured more toward maximizing the predictability of useful medications from the laboratory. The development of the new semisynthetic penicillins is a classic example of this new approach. By studying the structure of past successful drugs and by making proper molecular modification, the medicinal chemists have come to be remarkably successful in designing new drugs that provide the specific activity desired with a minimum of undesirable side effects. The activity of the new compounds can then be determined in vitro and in animal screens.

However, despite the seeming logic of this process and its wide acceptance as the most efficient means for the discovery and development of new drugs, it is also true that we can never know a drug totally when the only information comes from the preclinical screen. History teaches us not to be surprised if a drug is evaluated for one indication based on preclinical data and is accidentally discovered to have a particular activity in another therapeutic area.

The important point is that the medicinal value of all drugs—whether they are products of accident or design—can only be discovered after the drug has been evaluated in man. Only clinical investigation reveals the scientific and practical value of drugs. Thus the CDD must become the key factor in bringing to fruition a drug that might otherwise have been lost in the laboratory.

In sum, he will be responsible for directing the career of a new drug from the time it is first identified as having potential medicinal value through approval by the Food and Drug Administration. He must be a generalist responsible for structuring the sequence of events that will culminate in making a new drug available for general use and for overseeing the multiplicity of decisions involved in this procedure.

His tasks will include encouraging the transition of worthwhile investigational drugs from animals to man, deciding how best to determine efficacy in man, supervising the research that leads to a determination as to efficacy, and following through on the myriad details relating to such factors required for FDA approval as optimum dosage schedule, possible side effects and contraindications, and recommendations for use.

Perhaps his basic responsibility for some years to come will be to develop a more imaginative, sophisticated, efficient, and safer methodology for testing drugs in man at a far earlier stage in their development. In this way he could obtain a better understanding of the present animal screens, with a view to establishing a more precise correlation between the effect of a drug in animals and in man.

The emergence of the CDD has been slow, for the specialty is difficult, and places to train are few. To date, no one can "take a course," and even the pharmaceutical industry—the most logical "residency"—possesses only a dozen or so institutions whose activities are of sufficient breadth and depth for the student to develop properly.

In the past, too, the CDD has been almost nonexistent—not because he was not needed, but because the need was not recognized. There are still those who cling tenaciously to the idea that among the pharmacologists, toxicologists, clinical pharmacologists, clinical researchers, and other experts in the pharmaceutical area there should be no problem in finding those capable of handling the task of clinical drug development.

I do not agree.

True, the expanding twentieth century knowledge and technology has brought about a vastly increased number of specialists. The situation was accurately predicted by the prophetic Francis Bacon when he wrote, "For only then will men begin to know their strength when, instead of great numbers all doing the same things, one shall take charge of one thing, and another of another."

4

This is precisely what has happened: A wide variety of specialists has come along; they are exceptionally talented in their respective fields, and—almost to a man—they have not been exposed to the broad problems of clinical drug development. Today the growing complexity of research, the new legislation relating to pharmaceutical research, and the widening of public policy issues regarding drugs have all created an immediate need for the direction and guidance of a generalist with a workable knowledge of pharmacology and toxicology, some amount of medicinal chemistry and physiology, and, perhaps most important, an awareness of the temperament of society.

As the drug research process continues to become more complex, and the demands of consumerism more dichotomous, clinical drug development must of necessity become the critical specialty that can deal with the science of drug discovery and development and the politics that surround that process.

That is what this book is about.

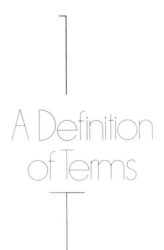

A Definition
of Terms

his compound is too toxic in certain animals to warrant consideration of a clinical trial in man." "Judging from the animal data we should aim for a dose of x mg in the human."

These are the often heard phrases that arise in the clinical use of drugs, no doubt due to subjective interpretations of some basic concepts involved in decision making.

Occasionally these phrases have merit, but as a rule they are based on individual interpretation rather than on the principles of drug activity. This chapter will examine some important concepts in drug development today, namely, toxicity, efficacy, margin of safety, and acceptable risk, because these concepts are extremely important in understanding the judgments people make about a drug.

Any discussion or attempt at defining these concepts can be rather perplexing and always elusive. They are by no means well-circumscribed scientific categories that can be given a weighted value. "The world is my idea," wrote Schopenhauer, and one suspects that these concepts are applied in the way individuals perceive them.

Rather than attempting to rigidly define the concepts of toxicity, efficacy, margin of safety, and acceptable risk, some salient features will be studied. Thus illuminated, hopefully these concepts will not be handled so cavalierly by those who are evaluating drugs.

Concept of Toxicity

The decision whether to evaluate a compound in man is more often based on the nature of the toxicity data than on the nature of the beneficial effect. Therefore, toxicity can be considered an important rate-limiting step in drug development today. It follows that this concept requires the closest examination and the most careful analysis.

What does "toxic compound" mean?

What do we mean when we say that "this compound is certainly too toxic to administer to man"?

Most, if not all, compounds are toxic. Therefore, to state that a compound is toxic is an exercise in tautology and adds little to the thinking process for clinical evaluation. Let us examine some common considerations for evaluating toxic substances.

A frequent error is to confuse the nature and degree of toxicity with potency. Potency is a quantitative term, and it expresses an effect that occurs *at a particular dose*. A drug that causes a toxic effect at 1 mg/kg is ten times more potent than a drug that causes the same effect at 10 mg/kg. The potency and toxicity of these compounds should not be confused, and the following examples may offer some clarification.

Compound A destroys 50% of the liver at 1 mg/kg, and compound B causes the same degree of damage at 2 mg/kg. Both compounds are equally toxic at the doses studied because they cause the same amount of damage. Compound A is, therefore, usually said to be more toxic than compound B; in reality, the first compound is more potent than the second and not necessarily more toxic. The wedding of the concept of potency to that of toxicity is a common phenomenon.

Other complications arise. Compound C causes hepatic damage at 2 mg/kg, but it might cause exactly the same type of toxicity at 4 mg/kg. Compound D, which also causes hepatic toxicity at 2 mg/kg, might in addition cause renal and myocardial damage at 4 mg/kg. Thus, the relative toxicities of both drugs change at different dose levels. Which compound is more toxic?

If compound E significantly lowers the blood sugar in a rat at 1.0 mg/kg and also destroys the kidneys at the same dose, this compound is more toxic than compound F, which lowers blood sugar at 0.1

mg/kg without affecting the kidneys, yet destroys the kidneys at 1.0 mg/kg. Although both compounds destroy the kidneys at 1.0 mg/kg, the first compound is considered more toxic than the second simply because the toxicity reference point is the dosage required to do something beneficial in the animal screen. This reasoning is indicative of the basic philosophy of the "art" and not the "science" of medicine. Both drugs are similarly toxic at the same dose, yet compound F is considered less toxic because the "good" it does occurs at a dose lower than its toxic dose, while for compound E the two results coincide. Scientifically, is this definition of toxicity really valid?

There are other considerations that affect decisions regarding toxicity. If a compound destroys 50% of the liver, is it more toxic than one that destroys 25% of the liver and 25% of the kidney? Which is more toxic: a compound that causes significant but reversible hepatic damage or one that causes moderate but irreversible hirsutism in the female?

Drug activity may be judged to have good or bad effects.* Bad effects range from sleepiness and allergy to cardiac arrest. Note, however, that an effect is labeled bad only in relation to the clinical situation. For example, drowsiness associated with a tranquilizer is considered an adverse effect if the patient is at work but a beneficial effect if the patient has difficulty sleeping at night. The bone marrow depressant effect of some drugs is considered beneficial for some types of leukemia, but harmful for certain types of skin disease.

TOXICITY VERSUS UNDESIRABLE EFFECTS   I personally would like to use the term toxicity sparingly and consider the undesirable effects of drugs in another light. However, the term is so entrenched that it would be practically impossible to discard it. Thus, adverse effect and toxicity will be used interchangeably here.†

Concept of Efficacy

Efficacy can be defined as the intended effect of a compound. Whereas some think of a compound as being either therapeutic or

---

* A third category of drug activity is judged to be neither good nor bad, for example, the nonesterified fatty-acid lowering effect of salicylates in a starving patient who has a headache and takes aspirin.
† For our purpose, a phenomenon such as anaphylaxis will be considered toxic even though it is not dose related and is idiosyncratic.

8

prophylactic, sometimes it is not known whether a drug is either one or the other. For example, what can be said about a drug that lowers plasma lipids. Is it prophylactic for heart disease, or is it therapeutic? The answer, of course, is that we do not know. The objective is to lower plasma lipids. The dose at which these are lowered is the efficacious dose—which might be prophylactic, therapeutic, inactive, or indeed contraindicated in patients with hyperlipidemia. The clinical parameter used to measure the lowering of plasma lipids (particularly during the early years of drug usage) is usually not sophisticated enough to determine whether this will benefit the patient, harm the patient, or have no effect at all.

Therapeutic or prophylactic compounds benefit the patient. Efficacious compounds do what they are intended to do, while hopefully being therapeutic or prophylactic. Penicillin is both therapeutic and prophylactic in certain infectious states; because of this, it is efficacious. In hyperlipidemia, nicotinic acid is efficacious; that is, it lowers lipids. But does it benefit the patient; that is, is it therapeutic or prophylactic? This is not known. Nor is it known if nicotinic acid is contraindicated for some reason, such as increasing the deposition of lipids in the intimal plaques.

In the subsequent chapters, the terms *efficacy* and *efficacious dose* will be used more frequently than *therapeutic* or *prophylactic dose*. The distinction between them is brought out here since it occasionally causes confusion and controversy among clinical investigators.

Concept of the Margin of Safety

As applied in modern drug development, the margin of safety is a great stumbling block.

A gross description of this concept is the toxic dose of a compound divided by the efficacious dose. The margin of safety in the animal is used as an indicator in deciding if any new compound should be administered to man. The closer the margin of safety is to 1, the less desirable that compound is, since this indicates that the toxic dose approaches the therapeutic dose. Conversely, when the efficacious dose is substantially smaller than the toxic dose, the ratio approaches infinity and the compound is considered more attractive.

Isn't it reasonable to assume that the higher the margin of safety is in animals, the more desirable the drug candidate for clinical evaluation in man? Isn't it sensible to choose from an animal screen a compound with a margin of safety of infinity instead of 1? Perhaps not. Unfortunately, the degree of acceptance of this premise is one of the great errors of modern clinical drug development. The predictability of a pharmacologic event from animal to man is not always reliable. The numerous variables in the biologic numerator and denominator preclude the complete validity of this test. This concept does have value, but it should be used with caution.

Concept of Acceptable Risk

What is an acceptable risk in people?

Is it related to the actual or potential good generated by a drug? Generally, the greater the projected good, the greater the risk one can take with a drug.

Most frequently, however, acceptable risk is a judgmental decision in which sociopolitical elements may override the scientific factor.

Take the vitamin-fluoridation comparison. Can anyone explain why there is such a substantial effort to restrict severely the general use of vitamins while at the same time a significant effort is being made to fluoridate our drinking water? Vitamins are essential to the critical metabolic process and have been given for years without evidence of toxicity except in cases of severe overdosing. Yet there are now indications that malnutrition in the United States is relatively widespread— even among populations previously thought to have adequate nutrition. Fluorine, on the other hand, is not a drug without significant toxicity. Clearly the actual or theoretical good is much greater with vitamins for increased nutritional status than with fluorine to prevent tooth decay.

Why wasn't saccharin removed from the marketplace along with cyclamate since both are similarly carcinogenic? Is the old standby, saccharin, somehow less of a risk than the unfamiliar newcomer, cyclamate?

The scientist and clinician must constantly avoid falling into the trap of inflexible thinking on this issue. They should be constantly aware that the risk-benefit ratio has a large element of the social— and, therefore, the unpredictable—in it. This ratio is rarely based on scientific thinking alone.

10

Perhaps the best advice would be to take a cartesian position and doubt any rigid application of the concept of acceptable risk until substantial proof is generated one way or the other. The truth is, as with foreign policies and lunar rockets, we will have to live with drugs without having all the answers.

2
Factors Involved in Drug Activity

Only when the CDD understands all the factors involved from the time an experimental compound enters the body until the time it leaves will the surprises be fewer and the results more understandable. The CDD should, in a sense, be a dilettante and have sufficient usable knowledge of drug events. He should know something about enzyme induction in order to recognize why the half-life of a compound is reduced with continued administration. He should then read and consult with the authorities on enzyme induction and understand more fully this empirical phenomenon. In this chapter we shall discuss just what does occur from the time a drug enters the human body to its exit.

A General View

For simplicity, events are usually described sequentially when, in reality, they occur in parallel. Illustrations depicting the life cycle of a drug in an animal or human invariably have absorption first, followed by metabolism, and ending with excretion. This tends to obscure the fact that all drug events are usually occurring at the same time. Frequently, a drug is in the process of being excreted long before absorption is complete.

Figure 2 summarizes the factors involved in drug activity. At a given point in time, one step usually dominates, even though all steps are occurring simultaneously. For example, if plasma levels continue to rise, then it is probable that more drug is being absorbed than

Factors Involved in Drug Activity

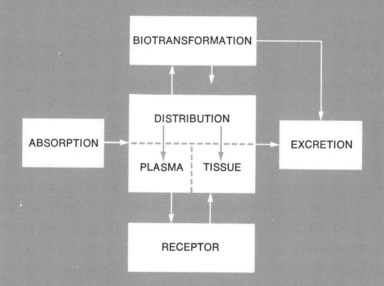

Figure 2

metabolized or excreted. It is important, therefore, to consider all these factors in relation to the ultimate action of a drug on its site of action, or receptor. Obviously, if a drug is not absorbed, it will not reach its receptor and no effects will occur—with the possible exception of local gastrointestinal effects, such as nausea and vomiting. If a drug is completely absorbed but rapidly excreted, then it might not be acting at the receptor long enough to bring about an adequate or indeed any pharmacologic effect. For any desired pharmacologic response, enough drug (concentration) must be present for a long enough period of time (duration) at the receptor. Then we hope for the best, since little knowledge of the elusive receptor exists.

Absorption, distribution, biotransformation, and excretion need to be discussed to understand the nature of drug action.

Absorption

Drug transport—either absorption from the gut to the general circulation or from the plasma to the cell—is based on the lipoid nature of the cell membrane, which is bound on both sides by protein. The principle is quite simple. Nonpolar (nonionized) compounds pass through lipoid membranes more easily than polar (ionized) compounds. Nonionized molecules that are sufficiently lipophilic actually appear to dissolve in the lipoid membrane and diffuse through and out into the aqueous medium on the other side. The greater the polarity, the less the chances of crossing the cell barrier.

This phenomenon is quantified by using the *partition coefficient*. This is done by obtaining the ratio of the solubility of a compound in an organic solvent to that in an aqueous solvent. The organic solvents commonly used are chloroform or octanol. Fat is technically difficult and impractical to use. The higher the partition coefficient of a compound, the more readily it will dissolve in lipoids, thus greatly enhancing its chances of crossing the lipoid cell membrane.

The great majority of present-day drugs are weak organic bases or acids which are largely, but not completely, ionized in solution at physiologic pHs. Nonpolar drugs usually cross cell membranes by passive transfer. This transport system requires little energy and is dependent on the physical properties of both the drug and cell membrane. The polar compounds, if they do cross the cell membrane, also

14

do so by passive transfer, but are quite dependent on the pK and pH gradient across the particular membrane.

Drugs can also cross cell membranes by a specialized active transport system. Active transport is highly specific, and high energy requirements are needed for the movement of a substance across the membrane. Foreign organic ions and natural substrates, such as sugars and amino acids, are transported by this system. Many of the antimetabolites fall into this category.

Concentration and solubility also play an important role with both nonpolar and polar compounds. If a highly liposoluble drug is not soluble in gastrointestinal fluids, then, regardless of its high partition coefficient, it will not be absorbed. As a rule, the higher the concentration of a drug in solution, the greater the absorption.

Is there a difference between the tablet or capsule form of a drug? For years it was assumed that it made little or no difference. Then a belief grew in drug circles that the absorption of a compound is largely dependent upon its dispersion in solution or fine suspension in gastrointestinal fluids. For this reason, the compound has been finely granulated and placed into capsules. There is an element of truth in this belief, but the exceptions keep increasing. For example, the diuretics triamterene and hydrochlorothiazide appear to be absorbed better in tablet than in capsule form (Fig. 3).

What about a difference between a patented drug and the generic form of the compound? Surprisingly, it has now been shown that the same chemical compound may differ in biologic behavior because of formulation. Chloramphenicol has become a classic example. The blood levels of branded chloramphenicol were significantly superior to those of generic chloramphenicol.[1,2] This is also true with oxytetracycline, among other drugs.[3,4] Though there is no evidence that the generic form is less efficacious as an antibiotic, there is a definite difference in at least one significant aspect of the purported comparable drugs.

Distribution

In evolutionary terms, a foreign substance entering the body is considered a threat. The organism immediately tries to rid itself of this intruder by a few basic mechanisms.

15

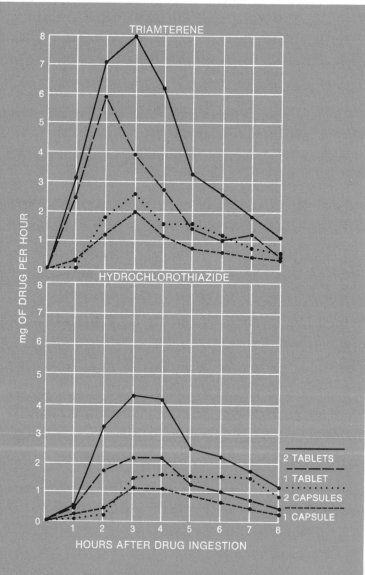

Figure 3 / The influence of dosage form on the activity of a diuretic agent. The curves show mean hourly rates of drug excretion in eight volunteer subjects after various dosage regimens. (From Philip J Tannenbaum, Earl Rosen, Thomas Flanagan, Archer P Crosley, Jr, The influence of dosage form on the activity of a diuretic agent, *Clin Pharmacol Ther* **9**:598–604, 1968.)

Generally, the body tries to make the drug more polar in order to excrete it.

The kidney tubule cells are lined by a lipoid membrane that permits the reabsorption of most nonpolar substances. This is why nonpolar drugs frequently remain in the body for long periods of time, whereas polar compounds are mostly excreted within 24 hours. Some have postulated that a nonpolar drug would remain in the body forever if it were not made more polar! With synthetic drugs, the living organism is confronted by substances that played no role in the evolutionary process. Converting these new nonpolar drugs to polar metabolites can be extremely difficult for the organism.

When a drug is absorbed, it can either be excreted unchanged, stored in depots such as body fat, bound to protein, or, if necessary, undergo biotransformation to a more polar metabolite. After absorption, a drug may pass through many fluid compartments, such as plasma and interstitial and cellular fluids. The greater the polarity, the greater the difficulty of passing into cellular compartments, thereby limiting distribution. Some well-established storage depots are plasma protein (usually albumin), bone, liver, and fat. For example, the antimalarial compound, quinacrine, after subacute or chronic administration to man will accumulate in the liver at a concentration many thousands of times higher than that in plasma.[5]

Fat as a depot for long-acting drug release is becoming more attractive to pharmaceutical scientists. Acutely loading the fat depot with a drug may give a slow constant release from the fat tissue into the circulation to the receptor for whatever effect is intended. Quinestrol, the 3-cyclopentyl ether of ethinyl estradiol, seems to act in this way. When administered orally as a single dose, it remains in the body for at least four months, since urinary metabolites can be found during this period of time and estrogenic activity is prolonged.[6]

But what if the body develops a toxic reaction to the drug and the only way to counteract it is removal of a substantial portion of body fat? This is why the development of an antidote to the circulating drug would be highly desirable before administration of the drug.

Recently, the polymer Silastic containing the drug has been implanted beneath the skin. This produces gradual drug release. If therapy needs to be stopped or if toxicity develops, it is easy to locate the Silastic and remove it. This experimental approach certainly looks promising.

17

Extensive binding of a drug to plasma protein, like ionization, can severely limit its distribution because the bound molecules cannot pass through cell membranes. The number of binding sites and the affinity factor of the drug to the binding site are important pharmacokinetic factors. However, there is no simple relationship between the extent or firmness of binding and the half-life or activity of a compound. A drug can be tightly bound and have a very short half-life.

The fact that a drug is stored can be either beneficial or detrimental depending upon the objective for the drug. If a high concentration in the plasma is desired, followed by rapid excretion, then storage depots will not help. If, however, a prolonged plasma or tissue level is wanted, then some form of drug storage can be extremely beneficial.

Biotransformation

If a compound is changed before being excreted, it is done by the process of biotransformation or metabolism. Biotransformation makes nonpolar compounds more polar to allow excretion. Detoxification does not always occur with biotransformation. In certain instances the metabolite is more toxic than the parent compound. The in vivo conversion of certain chemicals into active carcinogens is impressive evidence; indeed, this type of biotransformation could be termed "toxification."

In biotransformation the metabolites are more ionized, less lipid soluble, and, therefore, less likely to bind to plasma protein and tissue depots, including fat. Since they bind less and cannot penetrate cell membranes, they are excreted more readily. Because of the decreased ability of polar compounds to bind or be stored, it is not surprising that their metabolic rates are quite constant, whereas the metabolic rates of nonpolar compounds are highly variable.

Since many antibiotics are quite polar, their metabolic rates are also quite constant; by contrast, the majority of the psychotherapeutics are liposoluble, so their metabolic rates vary greatly. Since the variability of drug metabolism frequently can be correlated with the variability of efficacious response, we can predict, with reasonable certainty, the clinical response of antibiotics and other drugs that have a stable metabolic rate. On the other hand, the psychotherapeutics, which have unstable metabolic rates, also exhibit tremendous variability in onset of action and degree of efficacy.

The metabolic capacity of the individual is a function of many variables. Chloramphenicol unexpectedly caused mortality in children because it is metabolized at an extremely slow rate in this age group. It is probable that the hepatic microsomal enzymes are not at full capacity in the young. Now there are even indications that a diurnal variation exists in the liver's capacity to metabolize drugs; it is conceivable that a drug given at noon may be handled significantly differently than one given at midnight.

Drugs are metabolized along a surprisingly few pathways, attesting to the economic capacity of Mother Nature. Though drugs can undergo biotransformation in various tissues, this function occurs principally by enzymatic activity in hepatic microsomes. Changes that increase polarity are multiple and include such steps as increasing the number of carbon atoms or esterifying a carboxyl group. The principal pathways of biotransformation are oxidation, reduction, conjugation, hydrolysis, and exchange reaction.

The microsomal enzymes are distinctly different from those of intermediary metabolism. Only compounds with a high partition coefficient have accessibility to this biotransformation system, since there is no need to alter polar compounds that are already excretable. That the microsomal enzyme system does not metabolize the natural substrates of the body suggests that these substrates do not have access to the microsomal enzymes because of their lack of liposolubility.

Microsomal enzymes are quite flexible and readily adapt to different situations. When various phenols are administered to rabbits at low doses, they are primarily polarized by sulfate conjugation; when administered at high doses, however, they are predominantly polarized by conjugation with glucuronic acid.

Within species, the rate of drug metabolism varies notably. In man, the anticoagulant Dicumarol is metabolized with a tenfold difference in the rate among different individuals.[7] With some drugs, the disappearance rate from plasma is greater at lower rather than at higher doses. This can mistakenly be interpreted as a difference in the rate of metabolism when, in fact, it is a phenomenon of volume distribution.

There is another type of drug storage. At higher doses the drug can enter tissues like those of the reticular endothelial system before it is released. At lower doses the drug does not enter the reticular endothelial cells in great amounts and, therefore, is cleared from the plasma more quickly.

Excretion

Renal excretion of drugs or their metabolites is the predominant pathway of elimination of most drugs in most species. Liposoluble compounds, as we have seen, are reabsorbed by the renal tubules while lipoinsoluble compounds are not.

Radioisotopes have shown that biliary excretion of drugs is more common than previously thought. The enterohepatic pathway does play a predominant role with some important drugs. In rats, the enterohepatic pathway predominates in the metabolism of chloramphenicol. This compound is conjugated with glucuronic acid and excreted in the bile. It undergoes hydrolysis in the gut and frees the parent compound, which is subsequently reabsorbed. Strangely enough, this occurs to a much lesser degree in dogs and hardly at all in man.[8]

Organs of excretion such as the skin and lungs are sometimes important, but by and large they play only a minor role with most drugs.

A very good, but only periodically used, organ of excretion is the postpartum breast. During lactation many drugs, such as those used in the treatment of hyperthyroidism, can pass in large quantities into the milk and then to the breast-fed baby. From the time of conception to that of weaning, a drug given to the mother should be considered a drug given to the child—until proven otherwise.

The Receptor

Unfortunately, knowledge of the receptor has not kept pace with that of absorption, distribution, biotransformation, and excretion of compounds. Logistically, this is quite understandable, since it is difficult to locate the receptor and even more arduous to isolate it. Yet this is exactly what is needed to ultimately answer a multitude of drug riddles. How many similar receptors are there in rat and man? How much of a drug, in the same form, reaches each receptor for how long? These are the next significant questions in drug research.

Equally important is what occurs after the drug reaches the receptor. It is quite possible that opposite effects can be produced in man and rat from an equal concentration of an identical drug for the same duration for identical receptors. For example, hypoglycemia might occur in man and hyperglycemia in the rat. Therefore, in considering the mechanism of drug action, it is necessary to consider both *affinity* of the drug to the receptor and its ability to *induce* a response subsequent to the receptor occupation.

Most drug effects are thought to occur through three basic mechanisms:

1. Inhibition of enzyme systems or alteration of the specificity of enzymes

2. Alteration of the permeability of biologic membranes

3. Alteration of template molecules such as nucleic acids

Drug activity, while dependent upon chemical structures, also rests on physicochemical properties, such as van der Waals' forces, hydrogen and ionic binding, and spatial molecular configuration. These properties have only recently begun to get the attention they merit. Thus, on the basis of their spatial molecular similarities, distantly related chemical structures, such as estradiol and diethystilbestrol, can have similar biologic activity.

After reaching the receptor, drugs can act in three general ways:

1. *Agonist:* Drugs that produce a biologic effect after attachment to the receptor

2. *Antagonist:* Drugs that produce no effect after attachment to the receptor but block the action of another drug on the same receptor

3. *Partial agonist:* Drugs that produce partial efficacy (less than the agonist) after attachment to the same receptor as the agonist

21

Philosophically and scientifically these definitions are not strictly adequate, but they are a practical tool for viewing the drug at its receptor.

An agonist should produce an effect in proportion to its affinity or attachment to the receptor, while a partial agonist produces less than the expected response in proportion to its affinity to the receptor. Indeed a partial agonist can behave as an antagonist by occupying the same receptor as the agonist and thus preventing the latter from expressing its fullest capacity for efficacy. A true antagonist will occupy a receptor and not demonstrate any efficacy, but will completely prevent an agonistic response. An excellent illustration of the dose-response relationship between an agonist, partial agonist, and antagonist is shown in Figure 4.

The nature of a compound and its receptor is an expanding area in molecular biology; the expectations for this pioneering branch of drug research are great.

Enzyme Induction and Related Phenomena

So far over 200 drugs, usually the liposoluble ones, have been shown to produce enzyme induction. Enzyme induction occurs in the hepatic microsomes.

Some claim that it is difficult to quantitatively produce enzyme induction in individuals with cirrhosis equivalent to that in normal individuals, though so far the differences are not great. In man, phenobarbital increases the synthesis of microsomal enzymes which in turn increase the metabolism of the anticoagulant activity of bishydroxycoumarin, thereby reducing the plasma levels and decreasing the prothrombin times.[10] This effect decreases the anticoagulant activity of bishydroxycoumarin because the drug is eliminated from the body more rapidly. In the dog, tolbutamide induces increased enzyme activity to itself, thereby decreasing its hypoglycemic activity by shortening its presence in the body and its availability to the receptor. Tolbutamide does not do this in man, and probably, for this reason, tolerance does not occur in this species.[11]

The opposite phenomenon—that of enzyme inhibition—can also occur. Phenyramidol inhibits the microsomal enzymes that metabolize certain anticoagulants, thus increasing the anticoagulant response.[12] In this age of polypharmacy, the clinical investigator must be ex-

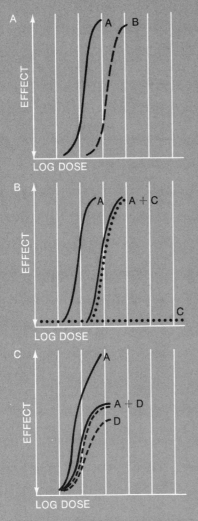

Figure 4 / Examples of dose-response curves of agonists and partial agonists. (A) Drugs A and B are agonists; they have equal efficacies, but A has 10 times the affinity of B. (B) Drug C is a competitive antagonist of drug A. It may have a high affinity but exhibits negligible efficacy. The degree of displacement of the curve for A in the presence of C depends on the concentration of C relative to its dissociation constant. (C) Drug D is a partial agonist. It may have an affinity of the same order of magnitude as that of agonist A, but its efficacy is less than that of A. The intermediate curve results if a dose of a mixture of A and D is administered. The exact shape and position of the intermediate curve depends on the ratio of the concentrations of A and D. (From HG Mautner, The molecular basis of drug action, *Pharmacol Rev* **19**:110. ©1967, The Williams & Wilkins Co. Reproduced by permission.)

tremely watchful for effects such as these. It has not been fully accepted that the action of one drug can be greatly enhanced by the addition of another unrelated drug. The average hospitalized patient on the medical service is said to receive approximately ten drugs during his stay, while the patient hospitalized for an extended period of time receives 18 drugs—a wonderful environment for enzyme induction or inhibition.

Phenylbutazone probably potentiates the anticoagulant effect of chlorophenoxyisobutyrate (CPIB) by displacing the anticoagulants that are largely bound to plasma albumin (Table 1). This could mistakenly be interpreted as enzyme inhibition if the problem were not carefully evaluated. Enzyme inhibition, however, is not at all a rare commodity. SKF525A, which has no known pharmacologic activity of its own, inhibits the metabolism of morphine, amphetamine, barbiturates, and many other drugs.[13] Although enzyme induction and inhibition are usually reversible phenomena, it can sometimes take months for the patient to return to normal.

There are many other examples of enzyme induction and inhibition and variations of metabolism within the species. The data indicate that with polypharmacy the phenomenon of enzyme alteration is probably much more common than we think. Therefore, this possibility should always be considered when the "unusual" drug event occurs.

The implications of the use of enzyme induction or inhibition in the treatment of disease stirs the imagination. As an extreme example, the carcinogen 3-4 benzpyrene, when hydroxylated, is converted into a metabolite that is noncarcinogenic. The human placenta of nonsmokers cannot metabolize 3-4 benzpyrene because of insufficient hyproxylase activity. However, the placenta of the smoking female is capable of metabolizing this carcinogen to a noncarcinogen metabolite because of increased enzyme hydroxylating activity. A somewhat heretical conclusion might be that smoking protects the pregnant female from carcinogenic hydrocarbons!

Drugs and the Receptor

Though most variations in drug activity to date have been attributed to the variability of drug metabolism among the species or to the phenomenon of enzyme induction or inhibition, there is also the

Table 1/Effect of "Clinical" Concentrations of Drugs on the Binding of Warfarin-^{14}C to Human Albumin

Drug	μg/ml	Warfarin-^{14}C (% Bound)
Phenylbutazone*	0	97.4 ± 0.5
	50	79.3 ± 1.1
	100	70.6 ± 2.8
	150	62.5 ± 2.3
Chlorophenoxyisobutyric acid*	0	97.4 ± 0.5
	90	86.8 ± 2.8
	180	83.6 ± 0.6
	270	75.1 ± 3.9
Phenyramidol	20	96.4 ± 0.7
D-Thyroxine	3	97.0 ± 0.6

* With increased concentration of phenylbutazone and chlorophenoxyisobutyric acid, the percent binding of these drugs to warfarin is decreased.

Source: HM Solomon and JJ Schrogie, The effect of "clinical" concentrations of drugs, *Biochem Pharmacol* **16**:1219–1226, 1967. Permission granted by Microforms International Marketing Corporation.

crucial factor of the nature of the receptor. In individuals in whom the anticoagulant bishydroxycoumarin is metabolized more or less similarly, there is a wider range of individual variations in the anticoagulant response than would be expected.[14] This is probably due to an intraspecies genetic difference in the affinity of the drug to the receptor. Also, like hepatic microsomal enzymes, the receptor can undergo some type of change when exposed to drugs. The administration of D-thyroxine to man increases the anticoagulant activity of coumarin-like drugs without any reported change in the metabolism of the latter drugs.[15] D-Thyroxine has been shown to increase the affinity between warfarin and its receptor almost threefold; this explains the increased anticoagulant activity.[15]

Thus, factors such as genetic disposition and other drugs can either increase or decrease the affinity of a compound for its receptor.

Beyond the Receptor

Continuous drug administration results in decreased efficacy for some compounds. Drug metabolism and the receptor are not altered,*

* This phenomenon is sometimes called *tachyphylaxis*.

25

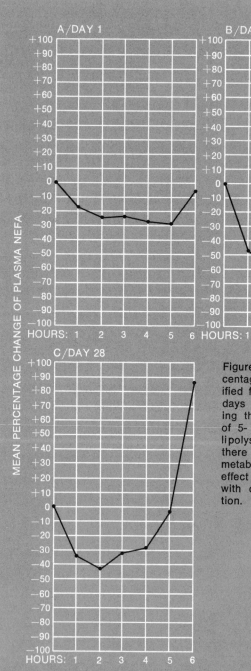

Figure 5 / The average percentage change of nonesterified fatty acids (NEFA) on days 1, 14, and 28, following the oral administration of 5- (3-pyridyl)tetrazole, a lipolysis inhibitor. Though there is no alteration in metabolism of the drug, its effect on NEFA diminishes with continued administration.

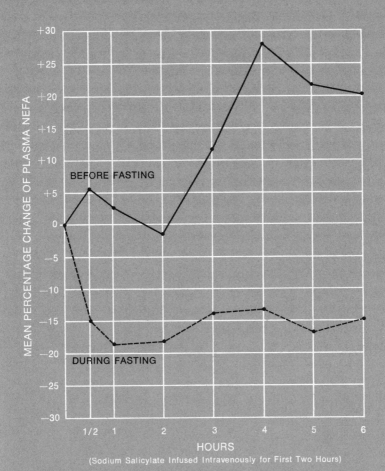

Figure 6 / The effect of intravenous sodium salicylate in obese patients before and during fasting. (Modified from SL DeFelice and SG Gilgore, A comparison of the effect of sodium salicylate on blood glucose and plasma nonesterified fatty acids in the fed and fasting states, *Amer J Med Sci* **256**(3):202–205, 1968.)

although the latter has not been as extensively investigated as the former. The lipolysis inhibitor, 5-(3-pyridyl) tetrazole, was given for a period of 28 days to determine its NEFA-lowering effect (Fig. 5). On day 1, the NEFA-lowering effect is quite pronounced. On day 14, the effect is diminished; on day 28, it is further diminished. A compensatory mechanism such as the phenomenon of vasoconstriction that follows hypotension might have occurred to produce this acquired resistance. One wonders if the so-called failures in human trials are due to compensatory changes beyond the receptor, rather than to the problem of the proper molecule getting to the proper receptor.

Age, sex, nutrition, and many other factors modify drug activity significantly. Yet, among drug researchers, these factors are usually mentioned briefly, are often dismissed as oddities, and are rarely pursued in depth. For example, usually the young animal is more sensitive to drugs because the immaturity of the hepatic microsomal enzymes results in a decreased capacity for drug metabolism. But there are exceptions to this. Ouabain is more toxic to the adult than the young guinea pig.[16] An exaggerated example of how the nutritional state can affect drug activity is shown in Figure 6. Sodium salicylate infused intravenously in the fed human volunteer has no NEFA-lowering effect. After a three-day fast, however, there is a pronounced NEFA-lowering effect that persists for at least six hours.

With more sophisticated clinical research, dramatic differences in drug behavior will probably be found between women and men, between the obese and nonobese, etc. These and other factors are discussed in the following pages.

References

1. Glazko AJ, Kinkel AW, Alegnani WC, et al: An evaluation of the absorption characteristics of different chloramphenicol preparations in normal human subjects. *Clin Pharmacol Ther* 9:472–483, 1968.

2. Martin MC, Rubin M, O'Malley WE, et al: Comparative physiological availability of "brand" and "generic" drugs in man: Chloramphenicol, sulfisoxazole, and diphenylhydantoin. *The Pharmacologist* 10:167, 1968.

3. Brice GW, Hammer HF: Therapeutic nonequivalence of oxytetracycline capsules. *JAMA* 208:1189–1190, 1969.

4. Blair DC, Barnes WR, Wildner LE, et al: Biological availability of oxytetracycline HCl capsules. *JAMA* 215:251–254, 1971.

5. Osol A, Pratt R, Altschule MD: *The US Dispensatory and Physician's Pharmacology*, ed 26, Philadelphia, JB Lippincott Co., 1967, pp 978–979.

6. Goodman LS, Gilman A: *The Pharmacological Basis of Therapeutics*, ed 4. New York, The Macmillan Co, 1970, p 1545.

7. Vessel ES, Page JD: Genetic control of Dicumarol levels in man. *J Clin Invest* 47:2657–2663, 1968.

8. Glazko AJ (discussion) in Williams RT, Milburn P, Smith RL: The influence of enterohepatic circulation on toxicity of drugs. *Ann NY Acad Sci* 123:122, 1965.

9. Remmer H, Merker HJ: Effect of drugs on the formation of smooth endoplasmic reticulum and drug-metabolizing enzymes. *Ann NY Acad Sci* 123:79–95, 1969.

10. Cucinell SA, Conney AH, Sansur M, et al: Lowering effect of phenobarbital on plasma levels of bishydroxycoumarin (Dicumarol) and diphenylhydantoin (Dilantin). *Clin Pharmacol Ther* 6:420–429, 1965.

11. Remmer H: Panel discussion. *Ann NY Acad Sci* 123:305–311, 1965.

12. Solomon HM, Schrogie JJ: The effect of phenyramidol on the metabolism of bishydroxycoumarin. *J Pharmacol Exp Ther* 154:660–666, 1966.

13. Axelrod J, Reichenthal J, Brodie BB: Mechanism of the potentiating action of β-diethyaminoethyl diphenylpropylacetate. *J Pharmacol Exp Ther* 112:49, 1954.

14. Solomon HM, Schrogie JJ: The anticoagulant response to bishydroxycoumarin: I. The role of individual variation. *Clin Pharmacol Ther* 8:65–69, 1967.

15. Solomon HM, Schrogie JJ: Change in receptor site affinity: A proposed explanation for the potentiating effect of D-thyroxine on the anticoagulant effect of warfarin. *Clin Pharmacol Ther* 8:797–799, 1967.

16. Wollenberger A, Jehl J, Karsh ML: Influence of age on the sensitivity of the guinea pig and its myocardium to ouabain. *J Pharmacol Exp Ther* 108:52, 1953.

3

The Comparative
Data Game

hough a primary objective of animal studies is to increase the predictability of a drug in man to as close to 100% as possible, there are many reasons why this objective cannot be fulfilled at present. First, there are multiple variables that occur between and within species from the time of a drug's administration to its excretion.

The Factor of Time

Any drug effect has both a qualitative and quantitative aspect; that is, a drug event occurs in a dose-duration relationship. If a drug is given to various animals at toxic dose levels over a six-month period, what correlation can be made regarding the comparative duration in man? What is six months of drug administration to a rat equivalent to in the life span of a normal human?

Table 2 lists comparative data for the life span of animals versus that of man. The table indicates that giving a drug to the golden hamster for one day is (in reference to life span) equivalent to giving it to man for 66 days. While this is mathematically true, in terms of duration, is it biologically true?

The duration of drug administration to an animal is extremely important, particularly when one considers that the average life span of the rat—the animal most commonly used in toxicology studies—is approximately two years, and the average life span of man is approximately 70 years. This essential difference is often overlooked.

Several other important factors are also involved in consideration of comparative data.

Absorption, Biotransformation, Distribution, and Excretion

If the course of a drug and receptor are similar in two different animals, then the predictability of drug activity from one animal to another should be greater. This is a sound hypothesis, and it is surprising how often these similarities do occur. But a slight change in the course of a drug can change this situation. A drug that looks interesting in the rat and monkey may have no activity in man because of inadequate absorption.

Man tends to metabolize drugs significantly slower than most animals; this is why he is commonly believed to be the species most sensitive to drugs. Table 3, which compares the half-life of papaverine, hexobarbital, antipyrine, and phenylbutazone in man and other species, lends support to this belief.

On the other hand, the anticoagulant ethyl bicoumarin acetate has a disappearance rate in man of 20%/hr whereas in the dog it is 3%/hr.[1] We cannot always operate on the premise that man is always the slower metabolizer.

Both the rate of metabolism and the nature of the metabolic enzymes can vary. Cats, for example, are unable to convert phenols to glucuronides, and dogs are unable to acetylate primary amines.[2] Since drugs can be metabolized along two or more pathways, the amount of enzyme involved becomes an additional and important variable.

Differences in the rate and nature of biotransformation can cause a drug to polarize less readily, which will affect distribution. This may result in the occurrence of more fat storage or central nervous system (CNS) symptoms due to easier passage across lipoid membranes, including the blood-brain barrier.

Both the comparable rate and the route of excretion are other important factors that can upset the degree of predictability with many drugs. Polarized compounds are usually excreted at the same rate in most species. The rate of excretion of liposoluble compounds, however, depends on the in vivo conversion to a more polar substance. The explanation in Chapter 2 shows how the interspecies polarization

Table 2/Life Span Relationship of Various Species to That of Man

	Percent of Life Span				
Species	Embryonic Period	Metamorphosis Period	Gestation Period	Lactation Period	Puberty
Golden hamster	2.5	1.3	4.5	6.1	12.6
Chinese hamster			4.6	4.6	17.6
Mouse			4.6	4.6	5.5
Rat	1.7	0.5	2.8	2.8	6.8
Guinea pig			4.4	1.5	4.2
Rabbit	1.2	0.2	3.6	2.4	10.6
Goat			4.7		7.5
Dog			1.7	1.4	5.8
Pig	0.5	0.5	3.2	1.4	5.9
Sheep	0.5	0.3	3.4		5.3
Cat			1.1	0.7	3.9
Monkey	0.6	0.2	3.1	2.7	20.0
Horse			3.6		4.0
Man	0.1	0.1	1.1	0.8	20.0

Source: Prepared by the Medical and Research and Development Sections of the Pharmaceutical Manufacturers Association, September 8, 1966.

rate can vary. The route of excretion of chloramphenicol is markedly different among different species. There is a predominant enterohepatic circuit in the rat that is not present in man. The continuous reabsorption of a compound may also prolong and increase the plasma and tissue levels, thus affecting drug activity.

Other Factors of Comparative Pharmacology

Many other factors in the animal screen affect the predictability from species to species. In most cases, these are probably related to absorption, biotransformation, distribution, and excretion.

The belief that young animals are more sensitive to drugs than the adult is supported by many examples. The reason usually given, though not always supported by data, is that the microsomal enzymes are not yet mature enough in the young animal to metabolize foreign

Average Life Span (Days)	Ratio Human Span to Animal Span
365	66
547	44
547	44
730	33
1,460	17
2,000	12
3,240	7.5
3,650	6.6
3,650	6.6
4,570	5.3
5,470	4.4
5,470	4.4
9,100	2.7
24,250	1.0

substances. For example, the liver of the newborn mouse is unable to metabolize phenacetin or hexobarbital, whereas the liver of the adult can. But here too there are exceptions. Ouabain, as we have seen, is more toxic to the adult than to the young guinea pig, and the older rat is more sensitive to myocardial necrosis induced by isoproterenol.[3] It is quite possible that microsomal enzyme activity can decrease with age. In man there may be a second childhood!

The greater sensitivity of children to drugs might be attributed too frequently to immature enzyme systems. Recent data suggest that variations in enzyme-substrate affinity may be the cause. There is also a common belief that infants excrete drugs more slowly than adults, which would explain some phenomena of increased sensitivity. Unfortunately, the data to support this belief are disturbingly few.

Sociology and genetic factors can also be responsible for some surprising reactions. Amphetamine and other CNS stimulants are

Table 3/Biological Half-lives of Drugs in Man and Various Animal Species

	Biological Half-life in						
	Man (Time)	Man (%)	Mouse (%)	Rat (%)	Guinea Pig (%)	Rabbit (%)	Dog (%)
Papaverine	100 min	100	8				35
Hexobarbital	360 min	100	5	39		17	72
Antipyrine	600 min	100	2	23	18	10	18
Phenylbutazone	72 hr	100		8	7	4	8

Source: Gerhard Zbinden, Experimental and clinical aspects of toxicology, in S Garrattini et al, *Advances in Pharmacology*, New York, Academic Press, Inc, 1963.

more potent lethal agents to mice when they are aggregated in one cage than when they are caged alone.[4,5,6] However, in a certain strain of mice, this phenomenon does not occur. Animals caged in a high-temperature environment are frequently more susceptible to the effects of drugs than those at normal or low temperatures.[7] Factitious hyperthyroidism in animals increases the toxicity of drugs and is perhaps related to a thermal effect.

Genetic factors can cause variation within the species. Primaquine, for example, causes hemolysis in glucose-6-phosphate dehydrogenase–deficient humans, a condition commonly found among African and Mediterranean peoples.[8,9] In the same population, no hemolysis occurs among those who do not have this enzyme deficiency.

The variability of the cortisone eosinopenic effect in different rat species is marked.

The antibiotic acetoxycyclohexamide is approximately four times less toxic in the male than in the female.[10] There are many other examples of genetic differences between and within species that affect drug behavior.

Environmental variables other than crowding can have a profound effect on body constituents. Care must be taken not to attribute them to drug activity. Decreased food intake can significantly affect the bone marrow of the rat and cause such changes as decreased promyelocytes, myelocytes, eosinophiles, and hemoglobin-containing erythroblasts. Table 4 shows some effects of malnutrition on various organs.

Diseases in animal colonies might be difficult to detect yet profoundly influence drug activity. Renal disease causing decreased drug excretion can, in some instances, easily increase the sensitivity of the animal to an otherwise well-tolerated dose. At autopsy, it may sometimes be difficult to be sure if the drug caused the renal change or if it was a natural phenomenon. This is one reason for control groups. If an animal loses weight, is it a direct effect of the drug or could it be that the bitterness of the experimental compound mixed with the feed is causing decreased food intake? There might indeed be a dual effect!

One must constantly beware of hasty, incorrect conclusions concerning a drug-event causal relationship—both in a positive and negative sense. Urticaria and exfoliative dermatitis do not occur in animals. If a rat had a headache, no one would know! Rats do not vomit and dogs always do!

The Litchfield Study[11]

The Litchfield study is mentioned separately because it is unique. The study involved a retrospective analysis of six unnamed drugs of dissimilar chemical structures that had been thoroughly tested in the rat, dog, and man. The drugs evaluated included an antibiotic, a synthetic antibacterial agent, a tranquilizer, a CNS depressant, a chemical that blocks the oxidation of alcohol, and a glucocorticoid. Comparative data of this sophistication are usually contained within the walls of the pharmaceutical community, inaccessible to most students of comparative drug activity. Some day, perhaps, more such information will be released for study purposes.

The Litchfield study tried to determine whether adverse effects (not efficacy) occurring in the animal screens could be predicted in man. Adverse effects are classified as signs or symptoms. A *sign* can be defined as any occurrence of an adverse effect that is not a symptom. A *symptom* is an adverse effect that is verbally communicated by the volunteer or patient to the physician. Symptoms cannot be detected in animals because of our ignorance of the languages of our evolutionary brethren.

The study was of a qualitative nature since it did not take into consideration the frequency of a sign, but simply its occurrence. If one sign occurred once and another ten times, both were given equal

35

Table 4/Organ Changes in Young and Adult Rats due to Malnutrition*

Age	Acute Starvation		Subacute Starvation
	Young	Adult	Young
Bone marrow	Decrease in cellularity +, mostly at expense of erythroblasts; atrophy of fat cells, increase of polynuclear neutrophile leucocytes +++	Decrease in cellularity +, mostly erythroblasts	Decrease in cellularity ++, hyperemia +++, edema +++, often hemorrhages
Spleen	Disappearance of lymph follicles and erythroblasts, swelling of reticulum cells +	Decrease of erythroblasts +	Disappearance of lymph follicles and erythroblasts, swelling of reticulum cells +
Testis	Inhibition of spermatogenesis ++, degenerative changes of the seminiferous epithelium ++	Interstitial edema	Atrophy +++, inhibition of spermatogenesis +++, desquamation and degeneration of the seminiferous epithelium ++
Adrenal gland	Decrease of sudanophil and doubly refractive lipids in z. fasciculata +++, delineation of z. glomerulosa indistinct	Decrease of sudanophil and doubly refractive lipids in z. fasciculata + to ++	Decrease of sudanophil and doubly refractive lipids in z. fasciculata ++
Liver	Atrophy and dissociation of liver cells + to ++, irregularity of nuclear size +	Atrophy of liver cells +, hyperemia +	Atrophy and vacuolization of liver cells + to ++, occasionally single cell necrosis
Kidney	Atrophy +, 2 rats fatty infiltration of tubular epithelium +	Fatty infiltration of tubular epithelium + to ++	Atrophy +, 2 rats fatty infiltration of tubular epithelium +

* *Key:* + slight, ++ moderate, +++ marked, z. zona.

Source: Gerhard Zbinden, Experimental and clinical aspects of toxicology, in S Garrattini et al, *Advances in Pharmacology*, New York, Academic Press, Inc, 1963.

Subacute Starvation	Chronic Starvation	
Adult	Young	Adult
Increase in adipose tissue +, atrophy of fat cells +, decrease of erythroblasts and increase of polynuclear neutrophile leucocytes + to ++	Increase of adipose tissue +	Increase of adipose tissue ++, one rat severe hyperplasia of immature white cells
Decrease of erythroblasts +	No changes; one animal (anemic) increase of extramedullary hemopoiesis +++	No changes; one animal (anemic) increase of extramedullary hemopoiesis +++
Reduction of mitotic activity +	Atrophy +; inhibition of spermatogenesis +	Atrophy +, inhibition of spermatogenesis +
Occasionally slight decrease of lipids	Unchanged	Unchanged
Atrophy and vacuolization of liver cells +	Occasionally atrophy of liver cells; irregularity of nuclear size +	Atrophy of liver cells +; irregularity of nuclear size +
Fatty infiltration of tubular epithelium + to ++	Atrophy +, one rat single cell necrosis of tubular epithelium	Unchanged, one rat single cell necrosis of tubular epithelium

weight. It was quite apparent that the predicted occurrences of signs in man were not very good. The comparative data for one of these compounds is given in Table 5, and those for all six compounds in Table 6.

37

Table 5/Occurrence of Signs in Three Species*

Signs	Animal
Low food intake Weight loss or impaired gain Adrenal, lymphoid, and muscle atrophy Lymphocytopenia and eosinopenia Hyperglycemia	Rat Dog Man
Myositis Gastroduodenal ulcer Bacterial invasion	Dog Man
Liver damage Anemia Neutrophil increase Polydipsia Polyuria Parasitic invasion	Dog
Purpura Localized fat deposition	Man

* The first group of signs was observed in all three species. The next group of signs was seen only in dog and man, but not in rat. The third group represents signs noted only in dogs and not observed or reported in rat or man. Finally, two findings occurred only in man.

Source: John T Litchfield Jr, Symposium on clinical drug evaluation and human pharmacology. Part XVI. Evaluation of the safety of new drugs by means of tests in animals, *Clin Pharmacol Ther* **3**:665–672, 1962.

If a sign occurred in both the rat and dog, the predictability that it would also occur in man was greater than if it occurred in only the rat or dog. This predictability was greater than 50% above that of chance alone. The same held true for negative predictions; that is, if the sign was observed only in the rat or dog the predictability that it would not occur in man was greater than if it occurred in both. The signs for which no prediction could be made are listed in Table 7.

Of the 89 different drug effects noted in the study, 33 occurred in man only. Some would consider these findings encouraging; others discouraging. What is clear, however, is that from a scientific point of view the data demonstrate that the ability to predict from animal to man is not very good.

Table 6/Incidence of Same Drug Effects in Rat, Dog, and Man

Sign	Number of Drugs
Low food intake	6
Weight loss or impaired gain	4
Anemia	2
Leukopenia	1
Lymphocytopenia	1
Eosinopenia	1
Atrophy	
Adrenal	1
Lymphoid	1
Muscle	1
Renal damage	1
Hyperglycemia	1
Sedation	2
Impaired reflexes	1
Ataxia	1
Decreased activity	1
Hypotension	1
Total	26

Source: Data from John T Litchfield Jr, Symposium on clinical drug evaluation and human pharmacology. Part XVI. Evaluation of the safety of new drugs by means of tests in animals, *Clin Pharmacol Ther* **3**:665–672, 1962.

The Primate as a Predictor

Are primates really better subjects for preclinical trials for drugs? After all, primates do behave more like man than do other animals that are customarily used in preclinical tests. Since primates look like man, perhaps their enzymes and receptors are similar to ours. The predictability from primates may be greater than that from rodents, but the differences may not be so great as is currently hoped by some. As one authority on drug metabolism has noted, "Alas, the patterns of drug metabolism are so different that one wonders whether the current enthusiasm for primate breeding should not be tempered. It has already been shown that ICI-33828 is metabolized 20 times more rapidly, and antipyrine, phenylbutazone, amidopyrine, and oxyphen-

Table 7/Signs Which Occurred in Man That Were Not Predictable from Animals

Diarrhea	Gooseflesh
Increased food intake	Fever
Localized fat deposit	Rash
Aplastic anemia	Pimples
Thrombocytopenic purpura	Dermatitis
Oliguria	Scarlatiniform eruption
Anuria	Urticaria
Edema	Bullous dermatitis
Cheilitis	Phototoxic dermatitis
Glossitis	Erythema
Stomatitis	Desquamation of hands
Thrush	Vaginitis
Gastritis	Bladder irritation
Proctitis	Purpura
Constipation	Nasal congestion
Trismus	Interstitial myocarditis
Chills	Bradycardia

Source: John T Litchfield Jr, Symposium on clinical drug evaluation and human pharmacology. Part XVI. Evaluation of the safety of new drugs by means of tests in animals, *Clin Pharmacol Ther* **3**:665–672, 1962.

butazone, 6 to 10 times more rapidly in rhesus monkeys than in man."[12]

It is conceivable, though, that the evolutionary development of enzymes and receptors in the primates might permit them to serve as surrogates for man. But primates are difficult to maintain in confined quarters, and the quantity of primates is not nearly so great as that of some other species, so it will be a long time before we shall know the extent of their usefulness. As another leading authority on comparative primate metabolism has stated, "At present most of the data indicate that the Old World monkeys usually mimic man from a biochemical standpoint more closely than do the New World monkeys. Among the Cercopithecoidea, however, the macaques would perhaps be preferred to some of the other Old World monkeys. Among the New World monkeys the *Aotus* or owl monkey seems to warrant more attention, and of the prosimians the bushbaby (*Galago crassicaudatus*) looks especially promising."[13]

Species-specific Toxicity

The term *species-specific toxicity* is frequently used to describe two types of events: (1) An adverse effect that occurs in certain species only and (2) an adverse effect that occurs in many species, but does so in a few species at doses substantially below the amount that causes the effect in other species. For example, dinitrophenol causes cataracts in chicks and humans, but not in rats and dogs.[14] Thus, the former are considered *specifically sensitive* to the drug. The intravenous LD_{50}s for histamine in rats and mice are 400 and 200 mg/kg, respectively, while in guinea pigs and rabbits the LD_{50}s are below 1 mg/kg.[15] Imagine, if penicillin were screened in guinea pigs and hamsters, it would be difficult to get it approved for use in the general population because of the species-specific toxicity it causes.[16, 17]

Frequently, the causes of species-specific toxicity are unknown, but in many instances the occurrence can be traced to one or more of the classic factors involved in any drug action. The clinical investigator is in a difficult situation when he is confronted with an apparent species-specific drug effect in an animal. He can never be sure that the sensitivity is only specific to that one animal—which makes it difficult for him to know how he should proceed in man, or whether he should proceed at all. The species-specific toxicity of a drug poses extremely difficult problems for the FDA—which usually leads to an unfavorable ruling on the drug.

Teratogens

Currently a drug is labeled teratogenic if it causes abnormalities to the fetus at doses that are nontoxic to the pregnant mother. If a drug is toxic to the mother and also causes congenital abnormalities in the fetus, it is not considered teratogenic by most authorities.

As a general rule, the drug or its metabolites should cross the placental barrier for a teratogenic effect to occur. The separation of the toxic-vs.-teratogenic effect is based on a differential in sensitivity to a toxic effect. The greater the difference between the lethal dose for the fetus and the lethal dose for the mother, the greater the probability that a drug will produce congenital malformation. Although this theory has wide support, there are insufficient data to prove or disprove it.

Fetal sensitivity to drugs such as thalidomide varies significantly from species to species and makes proper evaluation difficult.[18] In fact, in both animals and humans it is difficult to detect teratology at all unless it is obvious. The effect in the offspring must be detectable. If the IQ of the rat were significantly lowered in 5% of the drug-treated population with no other effect than this, it would probably escape detection.

The occurrence of abnormalities, including the resorption of fetuses, can vary widely in groups of animals within the same species. Since spontaneous fetal abnormalities are not uncommon in certain animals, such as the rabbit, the toxicologist must be constantly on guard against attributing spontaneous events in the fetus to a drug. Control groups sometimes do not help.

The predictive value from animal to man is certainly made more difficult with drugs such as 5-fluorouracil. There are two strains of pregnant mice that respond differently to this drug because of factors not at all directly related to the fetus. The maternal liver in one strain metabolizes 5-fluorouracil in a way that prevents teratogenicity; the maternal liver of the other strain does not do this, so teratogenicity occurs. If in routine screening the strain in which no teratogenicity occurs is used, then the clinical investigator might feel confident about the drug. If, however, it is screened in the sensitive mice, then the investigator would surely be much more apprehensive. Yet the situation is the same!

In animals, radiolabeled material can be given to the pregnant female to determine whether the drug will cross the placenta and enter the fetal circulation. Other sophisticated methods of drug measurement sometimes eliminate the need to use radiolabeled materials. Generally, drugs with a molecular weight of less than 1,000 appear in fetal blood[19], although there are exceptions such as the decamethonium salts.[20]

There is little knowledge regarding the predictability of the teratogenic effects of drugs in the human female. The timing of drug administration during pregnancy is equally as important as the phenomenon of placental transfer (Table 8). It is believed that most drugs

Table 8/Thalidomide, Period of Sensitivity

Days Postmenstruation	Malformation
34–38	Duplication of thumbs
	Paralysis, cranial nerves III–VI
	Abnormal pinna
39–44	Reduced and deformed upper limbs
40–45	Cardiac anomalies
	Duodenal atresia
	Gall bladder atresia
42–45	Reduced and deformed lower limbs
44–48	Aplasia of femur or tibia
About 50	Rectal stenosis
	Triphalangism—thumbs

Source: W Lenz, *Proc Second Internatl Conf Congenital Malformations,* London, International Medical Congress, Ltd, 1964.

exert teratogenic effects during the early phases of the gestational period when organogenesis is occurring at a rapid rate.

Since many women often do not know they are pregnant in the early stages of the gestational period, it is especially important to exercise caution when prescribing drugs. The current viewpoint is that women of childbearing age who are pregnant or capable of becoming pregnant should not take any medication unless it is definitely indicated. But this does not mean to avoid aspirin for menstrual discomfort. For other circumstances, what is necessary medication should be determined by the physician. Of course, this does not apply to women taking oral contraceptives; they can take many drugs without fear of teratogenicity.

Some believe that embryocidal drugs are embryopathic at sublethal doses. For example, aminopterin given during the first trimester of pregnancy causes abortion in the majority of pregnant humans; given later it results in congenital malformations in a substantial number of viable offspring.[21] Though the logic of this belief is supported by some data, there are enough exceptions to make it questionable.

It is interesting to note that compounds such as salicylates, hypoglycemic sulfonamides, insulin, steroids, and such consumables as caffeine and nicotine have been reported to cause congenital abnormalities in certain animals. But these claims are based on such high dose levels that their significance is questionable.

The detection of teratogenicity in both animals and humans is an area that needs further development. There are powerful social and political questions that are affecting research in this area, and it is unfortunate that the primitive technology for predicting teratogenicity from animal to man is of little help in resolving these questions.

References

1. Burns JJ, Weiner M, et al: The biotransformation of ethyl biscoumacetate (Tromexan) in man, rabbit and dog. *J Pharmacol Exp Ther* 108:33, 1953.

2. Williams, RT: Altered drug metabolism. *Ciba Foundation Symposium on Enzymes and Drug Action*. Boston, Little Brown & Co, 1962, pp 239–244.

3. Rona G, Chappel CI, Balazs T, et al: The effect of breed, age and sex on myocardial necrosis produced by isoproterenol in the rat. *J Geront* 14:169, 1959.

4 Gunn JA, Gurd MR: The action of some amines related to adrenaline—Cyclohexylalkylamines. *J Physiol* 97:453, 1940.

5. Hohn R, Lasagna L: Effect of aggregation and temperature on amphetamine in mice. *Psychopharmacologia* 1:210–220, 1960.

6. Lasagna L, McCann: Effect of tranquilizing drugs on amphetamine toxicity in aggregated mice. *Science* 125:1241–1242, 1957.

7. Keplinger ML, Lanier GE, Deichmann WB: Effects of environmental temperature on the acute toxicity of a number of compounds in rats. *Toxic Appl Pharmacol* 1:156, 1959.

8. Pannacciulli I, Salvidio E, Tizianello A, et al: Hemolytic effects of standard single dosages of primaquine and chloroquine on G-6-PD-deficient Caucasians. *J Lab Clin Med* 74:653–661, 1969.

9. Kalow W: *Pharmacogenetics: Heredity and Response to Drugs*. Philadelphia, WB Saunders Co, 1962, pp 104–113.

10. Pallota AJ, Kelly MG, Rall DP, et al: Toxicology of acetoxycycloheximide as a function of sex and body weight. *J Pharmacol Exp Ther* 136:400, 1962.

11. Litchfield JT Jr: Evaluation of the safety of new drugs by means of tests in animals. *Clin Pharmacol and Thera* 3:665–672, 1962.

12. Brodie BB, Reid WD: Some pharmacologic consequences of species variations in rates of metabolism. *Fed Proc* 26:1062, 1957.

13. Smith CC: Comments on comparative patterns of drug metabolism. *Fed Proc* 26:1044, 1967.

14. Robbins BH: Dinitrophenol cataracts; production in an experimental animal. *J Pharmacol Exp Thera* 80:264, 1944.

15. Papacostas CA, Loew ER, West GB: Studies on the toxicology of a histamine liberator, compound 48–80. *Arch Int Pharmacodyn* 120:353, 1959.

16. Hamre DM, Rake G, McKee CM, et al: The toxicity of penicillin as prepared for clinical use. *Amer J Med Sci* 206:642–652, 1943.

17. Schneirson SS, Perlman E: Toxicity of penicillin for the Syrian hamster. *Proc Soc Exp Biol Med* 91:229–230, 1956.

18. Report of the Commission on Drug Safety, Washington, DC: *Fed Amer Soc Exp Biol*, 1964.

19. McGaughey HS Jr, Jones HC, Talbert L, et al: Placental transfer in normal and toxic gestation. *Amer J Obstet Gynec* 75:482, 1958.

20. Baker JBE: The effects of drugs on the foetus. *Pharmacol Rev* 12:37, 1960.

21. Oliphant H, Nicholson MB: Cytoxic drugs in pregnancy. *J Obstet Gynec Brit Comm* 75:307–312, 1968.

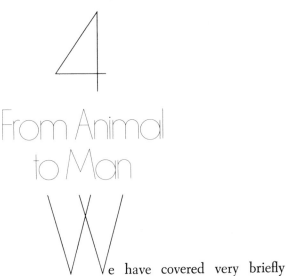

4

From Animal to Man

We have covered very briefly the issues involved in evaluating drug activity. We have seen that there are degrees of predictability and unpredictability in the areas of comparative efficacy and toxicity and that these are true not only from animal to animal, but, more importantly, from animal to man and from man to man. Indeed, the great evolutionary gaps in the biology of the species almost certainly a priori indicate that if there are gaps in the dexterity of the hand so also should there be gaps in the dexterity of the enzyme systems or receptor sites. It is a great credit to Mother Nature that there is an identifiable correlation from the animal screen to man; she must have had a very flexible initial design so that in subsequent evolutionary development much modification was not required.

While the correlation from animal screen to man can provide valuable information, it cannot be regarded as a strict guideline when taking an experimental compound from a nonpolitical creature to the most political creature of all.

In the next three chapters, we shall describe the history of a new drug from the time of its synthesis to its approval by governmental regulatory bodies. Here, we shall examine the rationale of animal screens in relation to clinical trials. The preclinical information derived from the screens includes (1) a demonstration of the compound's activity, (2) quantitative estimates of the acute lethal dose in several species, and (3) the nature of toxicity after subacute and chronic toxicity studies in rodent and nonrodent species.

Efficacy

The key that unlocks the door to clinical drug evaluation is primarily the fact that a compound has an effect in animals that is considered to be potentially beneficial to the human. When a pharmacologist finds a compound that can lower blood sugar in the rat, this drug may become a candidate for use in the diabetic patient. If this drug lowers the blood sugar in the diabetic patient but also causes a prohibitive adverse effect, it does not necessarily fall by the wayside. Instead, a medicinal chemist may synthesize other chemical analogues of the drug and pass them through the animal screen. If the synthetic analogues lower blood sugar, one or two candidates are chosen for further evaluation.

There are many animal screens that are used to predict the activity of a new compound. Some compounds are easy to evaluate; others are not. For example, an antibiotic can be more easily evaluated than an antidepressant, simply because in vitro and animal screens mimic the clinical entities of infectious disease sufficiently to provide parameters that have a high degree of predictability regarding human activity. With antidepressants, there are fewer relevant parameters, and those that are measured are vague and subject to broad interpretation.

Generally two types of screens for possible drug activity are used —in vitro and in vivo. In vitro screens are preferred since they are quick, reproducible, and inexpensive. Unfortunately, they are now only helpful in a few areas, such as infectious diseases. In vivo screens are time consuming, expensive, and subject to many variables. In addition, there are a number of reservations about their predictive value.

Few physicians are aware of the great amount of effort expended in the pharmaceutical community to create the design of in vivo and in vitro screens and to evaluate the findings. Does the thrombosis provoked by crushing the cerebral vessel of a rabbit with a metal clamp sufficiently mimic human cerebrovascular thrombosis to justify using this method as a screen for potential anticlotting compounds? What does platelet aggregation do to patients with vascular disease? Is it too optimistic to expect a beneficial effect from those drugs that were active in the screen? If too much logic is involved in evaluating the predictability of an equivocal in vivo or in vitro screen to the

47

human condition, will vital imagination and enthusiasm in the research organization be stifled? How does one select the one or two preclinical screens that have the greatest degree of predictability among the many? Are the cost and manpower effort prohibitive?

These are among the many questions that are asked in pharmaceutical research laboratories. They are particularly frustrating questions for the basic scientist since very few drugs reach man. The investigators frequently never know whether their ideas for the rationale of the preclinical screen are relevant.

Some enterprising scientists have attempted to routinely run compounds through a large number of preclinical screens, many of which are not related to the activity sought. The assumption here is that if enough screens are used, a more definitive pharmacologic profile of the compounds can be obtained, thus increasing the predictability of their use in man. For example, it is possible that a certain chemical series of efficacious antineoplastic compounds in people not only destroys rat tumors but also lowers uric acid in the monkey, whereas similar drugs that are inactive in man also destroy rat tumors but do not lower uric acid in the monkey. Knowing this, one can then predict a drug effect in man by an apparently nonrelated drug effect in monkeys. With this type of screen, computers can be used to detect patterns in the data that cannot be readily observed by the human eye. This approach deserves more serious consideration than it has received. It seems a logical next step in the evolution of a predictable screen.

Toxicity

Once the screening procedure has identified a potential candidate for clinical trials, the compound then undergoes animal toxicology studies. The nature of the projected use of the compound must be considered before designing these studies. If a compound is projected for use as a mild analgesic that will be available on drug store counters, it will undergo substantially more rigorous studies than a compound projected for use in phenylketonuria. The reason is that a large population, not under medical care, will not be closely supervised in their use of these drugs. If the animal experiments indicate that the risk associated with a new compound is great and the benefit is moderate, there is a tendency to discourage clinical development of the compound. This is especially true when another acceptable substitute is already available.

When a compound shows exceptional promise for an urgent medical need, an attempt is made to expedite initial toxicology work. In instances such as the treatment of terminal carcinoma, the classic recommended procedures of animal toxicology are cast aside, and the compound, after minimal animal studies, will be evaluated in man. Under most circumstances, the classic procedures of animal toxicology fall into two broad categories: acute toxicology and subacute or chronic toxicology.

Acute Toxicology

Acute toxicology experiments attempt to determine what effects are produced by a compound that is usually administered as a single dose. Nowadays, the LD_{50} is the criterion sought in acute toxicology experiments.

What is the LD_{50} and why was it chosen as a criterion in acute toxicology experiments? The LD_{50} is the median lethal dose, the dose of a drug that will kill 50% of the test animals. In most cases, the LD_{50} should be determined by both oral and parenteral routes to give the investigator some indication of whether the compound is being absorbed. Unfortunately, in some instances, only one route is used.

Commonly, two rodent and one nonrodent species are used for LD_{50} determinations. The dog or, occasionally, the monkey is usually the choice for the nonrodent category. This is an arbitrary decision, based on economic rather than scientific considerations; rats are cheap and gorillas are not. We hope that the rat, rather than the gorilla, is more like man in its response to drugs!

It is sometimes extremely difficult, or in fact impossible, to determine the LD_{50} in some species because of their capacity to tolerate a surprising number of compounds. Under these circumstances, it is quantitatively impossible to administer, particularly orally, the amounts required to produce a lethal effect.

Since the LD_{50} is a classic tool in acute toxicology studies, it is important to examine its significance. Some feel that the LD_{50} offers the clinical pharmacologist little information when moving an experi-

49

mental compound from animal to man. Also, certain data indicate that the nature of acute toxicity is not as important as that of subacute or chronic toxicity when considering this transition.

Nevertheless, the accepted procedure is to obtain an LD_{50}. Some of the reasons are as follows:

1. The LD_{50} is statistically easier to arrive at than an LD_{30} or an LD_{60}.
2. The LD_{50} gives the investigator a rough approximation of what dose level to use for man. From the LD_{50} other mortality doses can be easily found, for example, LD_{25} or LD_{75}. Acute studies provide more points on the dose-response mortality curve less expensively and with less time and effort.

   An LD_{50} frequently can be obtained by using 20 animals or less within a 24-hour period. One can then obtain a general knowledge of the slope of the mortality curve. As an example, in Figure 7, compounds A and B have the identical LD_{50}, but by examining the mortality curves at other doses, it becomes apparent that the LD_{50} is a misleading number. For compound A, the slope indicates that there is a broad range from the initial death to annihilation of 50% of the study group. With compound B, there is a very rapid transition from a no-effect dose to a 50% mortality dose. This becomes important in Phase I studies (see Chapter 5).
3. The LD_{50} can give the toxicologist an idea of what doses he should choose in the subacute or chronic animal studies.

The primary value of the LD_{50} and acute mortality studies is to aid the toxicologist in choosing a dose for subacute or chronic studies in the animal. Other than this, the LD_{50} is not really very valuable. In reality, a basic reason for its routine use is simply to comply with the customs of our scientific community and with government regulations.

Subacute and Chronic Toxicity

Subacute and chronic toxicity studies are more important than acute toxicity studies in considering the transition from animal to man.

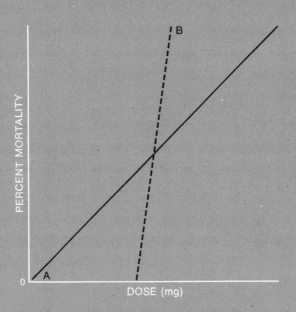

Figure 7 / The LD$_{50}$ is the same for compounds
A and B. The sharp no-mortality to mortality
characteristic of compound B should make the investigator more cautious in his dose progression
than with compound A, despite the same LD$_{50}$s.

The nature of the toxicity can be detected in subacute and chronic studies, whereas it is frequently difficult to make such a determination in acute studies. In most instances, the cause of death with acute administration of any compound is unknown.

A subacute toxicity study generally lasts for two weeks, but this period can also be considered a short-term chronic toxicity study. Many debates have centered around the transition point of subacute studies to chronic, but none has produced a conclusive answer. Actually, a determination of transition points is not pertinent to the clinical evaluation of a compound.

TARGET-ORGAN TOXICITY The primary purpose of all animal toxicology studies is to identify target-organ toxicity. In subacute or chronic studies, two species are generally used—one rodent and one nonrodent, frequently the dog. It is encouraging today that there is a tendency to add a third species, often the monkey.

With the help of the acute mortality data, three dose levels are selected for these studies: (1) No effect level, (2) some toxic effect but no mortality level, and (3) mortality level. By evaluating these three dose levels, a clearer idea of the nature of the toxicity can be determined. Not only can one evaluate the transition from no effect to mortality, but one can also determine the various changes in the animals during this transition. Toxicologists do surprisingly well in obtaining these levels through educated guessing. Frequently, a dose difference between each group is so great that a clear dose response is not obtained because of the lack of points on the curve. More dose levels would have to be studied to construct a curve as is done in the acute mortality studies.

During subacute and chronic studies, gross and microscopic pathology tests are done at intervals and at the termination of drug administration. In a 12-month study, some of the study group may be sacrificed at three, six, and nine months in order to trace and chart the evolution of the pathologic changes. The animals are also periodically examined for subtle changes that would not be normally detected by routine laboratory methods. One reliable method is to measure body weight. Since animals cannot verbalize feelings such as malaise or nausea, these must be detected indirectly by weight loss. Periodic eye examinations are also becoming routine, particularly since the possibility of ocular change has increased with more people taking drugs for longer periods of time.

When the animal data have been completed, the CDD faces a great moment of uncertainty. He now has the animal toxicology and efficacy data that tell him a compound is both toxic and efficacious. This means that the compound has some activity in the animal that can hopefully produce a beneficial effect in humans, that it is efficacious at an established dose, and that it has target-organ toxicity at certain doses along with a maximum tolerated dose in more than one species. If the compound is projected for use in women of childbearing age, teratology studies have also been done.

This multitude of data is supposed to enhance the safety of initial and subsequent drug evaluation in man. However, this is only partially true. Few data are needed to make a decision, and the accumulation of further data wastes valuable time that could be used in another way, as we will see in the next two chapters.

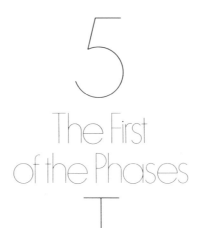

5

The First
of the Phases

The CDD is confronted with many problems when a new compound is taken from animal to man. A most critical one is that many of his early decisions must be based more on judgment than on fact; no matter how thoroughly the animal data have been compiled and analyzed, their predictive value is limited in the first and subsequent critical steps of clinical trials.

The introduction of a new compound to man is, for all practical purposes, an empiric phenomenon. The method used is the one that previously has produced the best data in the safest possible way. However, there is no single method and no precise guidelines. In fact, an unwritten law of clinical drug development is the more precise the approach, the more incorrect it is. To date, empiricism and broad guidelines established by medical authorities have proved the most satisfactory.

Three Phases of Clinical Investigation

Phase I

Clinical research takes the experimental drug from animal to man for the primary purpose of determining human tolerance. A substantial portion of this type of research is simply human toxicology studies. The objective is to cause adverse effects in small human populations in order to detect target-organ toxicity.

1. The initial dose in man should be extremely low, with estimates based on all the animal studies.

2. A modified geometric progression of the dose increments follows to a point just short of the maximum tolerated dose of the most sensitive animal species.

3. Fixed arithmetic increments are then given to cover the estimated range of the maximum tolerated dose of the most sensitive species.

4. Gradual modified geometric increases in doses are then given with periodic fixed arithmetic dose increments.

5. The drug is generally given until adverse effects occur.

Phase II

A compound is evaluated in reference to its efficacy; small populations are also involved.

1. Usually a dose closest to, but below, the dose at which adverse effects occur is judged to be the maximum tolerated dose in humans and is used to evaluate the compound's efficacy in Phase II.

2. Once efficacy is established at the estimated maximum tolerated dose, then lower doses are tested for efficacious activity.

Phase III

Large-scale studies are carried out once Phase I and Phase II data indicate that the experimental compound is worth serious consideration for use by the population intended. Essentially, large-scale studies are done to (1) determine whether the efficacy observed in Phase II will continue, (2) detect the select few in the population who are extremely sensitive or insensitive to adverse effects, and (3) see whether other effects not noted in Phase I or Phase II studies will be found. Ideally the dose that is farthest from the maximum tolerated dose but still as efficacious should be used.

Phase I

Initial Dose

In selecting an initial dose for Phase I studies, a small fraction of the maximum tolerated dose of the subacute or chronic animal toxicity studies in the most sensitive species is chosen. As a rule, the information obtained from acute toxicity studies is not sufficiently meaningful to be a guideline for selecting an initial dose.

In clinical research, man is considered the most sensitive species; therefore, data from the most sensitive animal species in the chronic toxicity studies should serve as a guideline to man. This policy is based on social or moral judgments rather than on scientific ones. The rationale is if man is the most sensitive species, then using the most sensitive animal species will increase the safety factor for humans.

Indeed, the classic darwinian might have a scientific argument to support this position. With the evolution of intellect in man, he has not undergone sufficient biologic evolution. He has learned by observation that certain substances are toxic and others nontoxic. Thus, early in his existence, his enzyme system did not have to adapt to the toxic challenges of his environment. Since animals lack the intellect of man, however, their enzyme system had to evolve. Those animals who could not adapt were destroyed, and, through natural selection, the ones that could adapt and develop flexible detoxifying systems survived. This hypothesis may or may not be justifiable. But even if it is agreed that man is the most sensitive species, arguments will invariably arise over the interpretation of this position.

When viewing the animal data two factors should always be kept in mind: (1) How long the drug was given to the animal, and (2) what is the nature of the toxicity. For instance, rats tolerate a compound given daily for a period of one year at 1 mg/kg, and monkeys tolerate the same compound under the same condition at 10 mg/kg. The rat is then considered the most sensitive species and will serve as the point of reference to man.

Since 1 mg/kg was the maximum tolerated dose in the rat, then a low percentage of that dose will be chosen for the initial dose in man. How low should it be? No scientific answer is available except that it should be absurdly low. If the drug is projected for short-term use in man—a period of one or two days—then a larger fraction of the maximum tolerated dose may sometimes be used for the initial dose. However, if the drug is to be given to man for a substantially longer period of time, the percentage of the maximum tolerated dose will be smaller.

If one wants to give a compound to man for one day, what should the point of reference be? The two-week toxicity study with a maximum tolerated dose of 100 mg/kg or the one-year study with a maximum tolerated dose of 1 mg/kg? The selection of the initial dose, clearly, must also consider the length of the animal study.

When selecting an initial dose, remember that it is not always possible to quantify the nature of the toxicity. Consider the following example. Two drugs are administered to rats at a dosage of 1 mg/kg over a six-month period. One drug causes a slight weight loss while the other causes hepatocellular destruction, nephrotoxicity, and cardiac necrosis. At 0.5 mg/kg, however, both drugs cause no toxicity. Whereas the estimated maximum tolerated dose for both drugs is 0.5 mg/kg, one would be more inclined to use a smaller percentage of the maximum tolerated dose of the compound that caused liver, kidney, and cardiac toxicity. Some will argue against this reasoning, but they should wait until they can prove their point.

What is an extremely low dose? What dose can be estimated from the subacute or chronic animal studies that will be considered almost 100% safe for the initial trial in man? Many decisions involve only qualitative phenomena, and mathematical formulas deal only with quantitation. There is no particular equation to solve this problem, although the search for one still persists. It is largely a matter of judgment.

If a compound causes slight weight loss at 100 mg/kg, but no adverse effects at 50 mg/kg for a period of over six months in the most sensitive species, then certainly it would seem reasonable to choose a dose of 0.5 mg/kg as the initial dose in man. This decision is based on the judgment of those experienced in drug research.

Dose Progression

Once the initial dose is selected, it is increased progressively to the stage where adverse effects occur. This procedure allows identification of target-organ toxicity in the human and also establishes an idea of the upper limit of the safe dose range. With some compounds, however, it is not always necessary to reach a toxic dose in humans. This is frequently the case with antibiotics where there may often be sufficient preclinical information to estimate the efficacious dose on the basis of blood levels. Because of variations in pharmacokinetics, though, this approach may not be ideal. The overreliance on blood levels as a predictor of drug activity has probably created a situation of underdosing with antibiotics. The very fact that there are significant numbers of therapeutic failures with antibiotic therapy indicates that not enough drug is being given even if the blood levels are higher than the MIC.

After the initial dose has been administered daily to volunteers for a short period of time, usually from one to three days, increments of the dose are then administered. Based on the available animal data, the progressive doses can be estimated through one of four procedures.

FIXED ARITHMETIC DOSE PROGRESSION Although this method is basically unsatisfactory, it is considered by some that fixed arithmetic progressions are generally too conservative and not realistic. If a dose increment of 0.1 mg/kg to 0.2 mg/kg is made in the initial progression, it is double the original dose and a significant increment. If a dose of 5 mg/kg is reached in man and there are not adverse effects, it was necessary to take 50-dose progression steps to reach this point, and the next increment would be 5.1 mg/kg!

FIXED GEOMETRIC PROGRESSION This progression is extremely attractive to those who are mathematically inclined, but not to those who are realistic drug researchers. Its basic defect is that the dose increments are too conservative in the initial progression steps and much too large during the later steps. In Table 9, a fixed multiplier of 2.0 of the initial dose has been arbitrarily chosen as an example. If one assumes that the initial dose is 10 mg, then the following increments are quite conservative up to, perhaps, step seven. From 7 to 10 the increments are too large, particularly if one is dealing with the possibility of serious toxicity. Those who prefer formulas for the study of drugs in Phase I will be hard pressed to justify their position. For, in this situation, they would have to look at the animal data and then choose a multiplier of 1.2, 1.5, or 2.0. This is indeed a difficult task in practically every case.

58

Table 9/Arbitrary Dose Progression Curves

Steps	Fixed Geometric Dose*	Function of a Line		
1	10	10†	10‡	10¶
2	20	20	30	50
3	40	40	80	210
4	80	60	190	740
5	160	100	390	2,200
6	320	150	730	5,300
7	740	200	1,200	11,000
8	1,480	250	1,700	19,000
9	2,960	280	2,200	27,000
10	5,920	310	2,480	33,000

* Assuming an initial dose of 10 mg with a fixed multiplier of two.

† Assuming an initial dose of 10 mg with an initial increment that is twofold.

‡ Assuming an initial dose of 10 mg with an initial increment that is threefold.

¶ Assuming an initial dose of 10 mg with an initial increment that is fivefold.

FUNCTION OF A LINE   In this procedure, a line is plotted on semi-log paper from the starting increment against the number of step-doses desired in the trial period. The log of the multiplier is on the ordinate and the number of steps desired is on the abscissa (in this example it is 10). The ordinate and abscissa are the same as the fixed geometric progression line. In Table 9, the initial increment is 2.0, or twice the initial dose, and the number of steps is 10. This approach also presents many problems, among them that of determining how many steps should be taken in Phase I. This, of course, cannot be determined from animal studies. Also, the increments in the latter part of the dose progression are extremely small, making this type of dose progression impractical, particularly with compounds that are well-tolerated at high dose levels.

EYE-BALLING   Here, a clinical pharmacologist reviews the data in its entirety—including structure, pharmacology, toxicology, metabolism, and species differences—and then decides what a safe progression would be. While this method is considered subjective, experience does not confirm this. "Eye-balling" is actually more of an objective-subjective approach since all the dosing in animals, along with all other data, are considered *before* estimating a safe dose progression.

There is nothing mysterious about eye-balling animal data and then constructing a plan for Phase I dose progressions. Admittedly, this approach is not readily accepted because it cannot be directly taught. Yet it is similar to auscultation of the heart: One can read about cardiac sounds in the finest medical texts, but cannot truly know them until the stethoscope has been used repeatedly. It takes many trials with many drugs before an investigator acquires a "feel" for the technique of creating a safe dose progression. Today, only a handful of clinical pharmacologists possess the art involved in this technique.

Those who favor the eye-balling technique use a modified geometric and fixed arithmetic progression. In this procedure, once geometric progression begins and a dose is reached that is just short of the maximum tolerated dose of the most sensitive species, a fixed arithmetic progression may then be followed through the estimated range of that dose. The reason, again, is based on the rationale that man is the most sensitive species. When the maximum tolerated dose of the most sensitive species is reached in man, then man, too, should be experiencing adverse effects. Therefore, dose increments should be conservative, that is, arithmetic. If after successive arithmetic increases, the level reached is well beyond the animal maximum tolerated dose, then it is assumed that man is not the most sensitive species and a modified geometric progression can again be started. If no adverse effects occur during this modified geometric progression it is wise to level off periodically to moderate arithmetic progressions. This is done in an attempt to minimize the impact of toxicity.

In Phase I studies, dose progressions are usually carried out until adverse effects occur. This immediately locates the target-organ toxicity in a small population before carrying out studies in larger groups. At a dosage of 1 mg, the incidence of adverse effects with a particular compound would be 0.1% and might not be detected in a small population study which is usually less than 100 volunteers and frequently less than 50. At a dosage of 10 mg, however, the incidence of the same adverse effect might be 25% and can usually be detected in a small population. Determining the toxic dose in Phase I also facilitates optimal dose selection for Phase II studies.

Usually, Phase I studies are terminated when significant adverse effects occur, although not necessarily, since some adverse effects disappear with continued drug administration. A dose that is just below the minimum adverse effect level is then estimated to be the maximum tolerated dose; at, and up to, this level no adverse effects are expected to occur. Choosing the estimated maximum tolerated dose is a matter of judgment and, therefore, is sometimes difficult to determine.

Is it the increment or duration of the dose that causes the adverse effect? For example, the dose of an experimental compound is raised every week for a period of four weeks and elevated SGOTs occur at the end of the fourth week. What is the responsible factor? Either it is the increase in dosage from the third to fourth week or the duration of drug administration and not the increment in dosage. Then one is forced to make an educated guess as to what a tolerated dose will be over a period of a month. Most, but not all, adverse effects occur within the first six weeks of drug administration. Some insidious effects such as eye changes usually take longer to occur. This must always be considered when the compound is being investigated for chronic administration.

Adverse Effects

Since the thalidomide tragedy, the public and the pharmaceutical industry have focused intensely on the phenomenon of undesired drug effects. Yet it is difficult to construct a scientific classification of adverse effects. Some investigators use the term "side effects" to describe findings such as nausea and vomiting and "toxicity" to describe something objective such as elevated transaminases. These classifications are convenient, but they tend to mislead the investigator into believing that the two types of effects are different when, in reality, they frequently are not. A volunteer with side effects of nausea and vomiting may have developed a gastric ulcer, which is indeed toxicity. The term "side effects" is then used as an excuse for describing adverse effects that cannot be measured quantitatively, either because no measurement technique exists or because a technique is impractical under the circumstances of the study. It is unfortunate, indeed, that in clinical pharmacologic circles toxicity is often viewed as being much more serious than side effects.

One might question the rationale of purposefully causing adverse effects in humans. Is this procedure actually necessary, or is it possible to choose a nontoxic dose at a fifth or sixth progression and then test for efficacy? With some compounds this is done—and even overdone! But with most compounds this should not be the usual procedure. It cannot be emphasized strongly enough that despite the thoroughness of an animal screen, predictions from animal data to man are not always reliable.

A striking example is the rodenticide norbormide. This compound is extremely toxic to certain species of rodents (in the rat the LD_{50} is 2.5 ± 0.5 mg/kg),[1] but it is much less toxic to other laboratory species (in the monkey the LD_{50} is greater than 1,000 mg/kg)[2] and to man.[2] The initial dose for this compound, based on the customary fraction of the LD_{50} in the most sensitive species, would be one-six-hundredth of 2.5 mg/kg, or the extremely low dose of 0.0042 mg/kg. The probability is small that this dose or even ten times this dose would be sufficient to cause a detectable effect in the human. It would take years to screen the compound for efficacy in the human if arbitrarily 0.1, 0.2, 0.4, 0.8, or 1.0 mg/kg doses were used to test for activity in man.

The point is to proceed to adverse effects and choose the maximum tolerated dose; if the drug is not efficacious at this dose then you know you cannot go any higher and the compound is essentially dead as a clinical candidate. This procedure saves much time and will bring the benefits of drug activity to man much sooner.

Phase I studies are usually done in prison populations. The advantages of studying a compound in any institutional population are significant. Volunteers are easier to observe and work with, and laboratory studies can be carried out on schedule. It is almost impossible to match this environment in any other clinical situation. Furthermore, inmates are currently one of the few groups that have expressed an interest in participating in medical research. Their motivation in volunteering is complex and involves the circumstances of the prison environment. A major factor (besides remuneration) contributing to the willingness of inmates to participate in research is their desire to participate in a socially acceptable task.

The social forces that influence inmates to volunteer, however, will inevitably affect the outcome of clinical studies. Often inmates will not report adverse effects for fear of being dropped from the study and thereby losing remuneration and social privileges. The investigator must gain their confidence and assure them that they can always take part in future studies; otherwise they may not speak freely.

There are still other disadvantages in carrying out studies in institutional populations. Certain abnormalities, such as transient fever, skin eruptions, hepatic and hemopoietic changes, frequently occur spontaneously in these groups and are often attributed to the experimental drug if the volunteers are participating in a study when the changes occur. (Parenthetically, it is interesting to note that these changes are rarely attributed to aspirin. I have heard of one observation where elevated transaminases occurred more frequently with a placebo than in groups treated with several drugs over a period of time in a particular prison—which suggests that drugs are hepatoprotectants! Many clinical pharmacologists have seen periodic elevations of blood parameters during drug administration which frequently return to normal level despite the continued administration of drug.)

There is also the occurrence of endemic diseases, probably of viral origin, that cause nausea, vomiting, fever, lymphocytosis, and many other manifestations. If these occur during a Phase I study, it is difficult not to implicate the drug. To avoid this, a controlled study should be run with a placebo and the experimental drug.

How can the investigator be prepared to detect any undesirable change? First, he has the animal toxicology data and some idea of the target-organ toxicity in various species. While the predictive value of the animal data is not 100%, the toxicity correlations are often sufficient. If data are available, the clinician must consider the nature of the toxicity in past experience with compounds in a similar chemical series and be thoroughly aware of the effects in animals and in humans. Thus, if a folic acid antagonist causes bone marrow depression in four species, one should expect the appearance of myelocytes in the blood followed by bone marrow depression in man, if the drug is pushed sufficiently. If, on the other hand, one encounters moon facies and the buffalo hump syndrome with a new steroid this should not be surprising just because steroids do not cause these effects in animals. A helpful guide is that the more common types of adverse effects are associated with the liver, bone marrow, skin, and gastrointestinal tract.

In Phase I studies significant, irreversible toxicity seldom comes on

63

suddenly. Volunteers are seen often, sometimes every day, and a physician is on call around the clock. Blood tests along with other types of measurements are done frequently in the initial phases and periodically thereafter. Adverse effects are almost always detected before they become a threat to the volunteer. Man's ability to communicate his feelings is a great asset in avoiding adverse effects. Since animals cannot verbalize, toxicologists must increase the dose until objective toxicity occurs. Perhaps the fact that man can verbalize the oncoming of adversity has contributed to his reputation as the most sensitive species. There are many pitfalls in trying to evaluate all the human adverse effects.

Here, we shall just briefly describe another important part of Phase I work—drug metabolism studies. At very low doses, experiments are run in man to determine whether biotransformation is occurring and the nature of the pattern of excretion. The results can then be compared to the metabolism studies in animals. If in the dog and the rat the experimental compound is hydroxylated and in man it is carboxylated, then the prognosis that the drug will be active in man is not as good. This is particularly true if it is the hydroxylated metabolite that is the active moiety in the animal screen.

Phase I is a fascinating stage in clinical drug development that has multiple ramifications. While some medical spokesmen view Phase I studies as being extremely dangerous, this is simply not true. These studies are usually quite safe when carried out properly. What is needed is more interest on the part of the physician if our progress is not to be greatly retarded.

References

1. Roszkowski AP: The pharmacological properties of norbormide, a selective rat toxicant. *J Pharmacol Exp Ther* 149:288, 1965.

2. Roszkowski AP: Comparative toxicity of rodenticides. *Fed Pro* 26:1082, 1967.

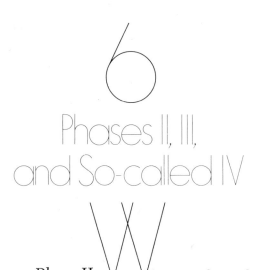

6
Phases II, III, and So-called IV

Phase II: When is a drug a legitimate candidate for serious consideration as a possible therapeutic or prophylactic tool in the general population? Phase II attempts to define this by determining (1) drug efficacy, (2) its margin of safety, and (3) other characteristics of the drug.

Unfortunately some of the questions that are raised in early Phase II studies must be answered initially through educated guessing. Was the unexpected occurrence of an adverse effect due to an unexpected prolonged half-life of the experimental compound found in Phase I, or was it due to the presence of a different metabolite detected by some form of chromatography? Is man more like a rat or a monkey in relation to the nature of toxicity and drug metabolism? If he is more like a rat than a monkey, can we expect the efficacious and/or toxic dose to be within the range seen in the rat rather than the monkey? Will the target-organ toxicity be the same? Frequently, some of the answers to these and other questions are not available until Phase II studies are completed.

The efficacy of a compound must be examined in as many aspects as possible; it is not just whether a drug is effective, but to what degree —20%, 30%? How does it compare to other compounds or a placebo? In the initial Phase II trial, *usually* the estimated maximum tolerated dose should be chosen to test for efficacy. As we have seen, in evaluating efficacy it is generally difficult and more often impossible to choose a determined dose for man from the animal data. But there are occasional exceptions.

ICI-33828 is an exemplary drug that demonstrates that blood levels can have predictive value.[1] This compound inhibits pituitary gonadotropic hormone secretion at widely varied doses in different species up to a 200-fold variation. Yet, despite the wide variation, the drug shows its inhibitory response at the same plasma concentration of 3 $\mu g/ml$, which was attained in each species at different varied doses. Antibiotics such as the tetracyclines have some predictive value from animal to man based on both blood levels and dose-weight relationship. Even in these cases, though, there are factors that make 100% predictability difficult. With a number of anticancer drugs, the dose that causes toxicity in the dog, mouse, hamster, rat, monkey, and man is similar when based on body surface area. But there is little correlation based on milligram per kilogram dosage.

Sufficient efficacious activity sometimes occurs at the maximum tolerated dose so that the drug candidate appears to be useful to the general population. If the maximum tolerated dose is too near the dose that causes serious adverse effects, then its use is questionable. In these cases, the dose is substantially lowered and efficacy studies are then repeated. There is no reason why multiple dose levels below the maximum tolerated dose cannot be studied simultaneously, provided, of course, that it is practical. The objective is to lower the dose as much as possible below the maximum tolerated dose without losing the desired activity.

It may be difficult and often impossible to titrate an optimal dose in a sophisticated manner because of the nature of the Phase II screen. If a compound was postulated to be effective against diabetic retinopathy, the maximum tolerated dose would arbitrarily be selected as the therapeutic or prophylactic dose since it would take a rather long time to evaluate any kind of activity at any particular dose level. If adverse effects occur, then the dose would be lowered and the study continued. When there are sufficient accessible populations available and when the activity of the compound can be determined without great difficulty and within a short period of time, then a thorough attempt to establish a margin of safety should be made. Unfortunately, many compounds are not tested under these circumstances.

By the completion of Phase II, it should be possible to make a reasonable judgment regarding the degree of efficacy at a particular dose and the nature of adverse effect at a particular dose. Whether or not further large-scale studies will be carried out rests on the consideration of these factors, all of which can be summed up in the concept of the risk-benefit ratio.

The Determination of Efficacy

It is the sad paradox of clinical drug development that more time and mental effort are expended on preclinical studies than on Phase II studies. While Phase I studies have become much more sophisticated, Phase II studies lag behind despite the overwhelming fact that the critical question is whether a compound is efficacious in the human, and to what degree and why. This must change. The ultimate value of a compound is its clinical efficacy, and the determination of efficacy is the rate-limiting step in clinical drug development. Therefore, in Phase II studies the proper questions must be asked and the experiment designed to answer these questions. This involves long hours of reading all the available data on the drug candidate, thoroughly reviewing the literature on related drugs, studying the conditions for which they are effective, and conferring with authorities in the field.

Case report forms should be designed to answer all of the questions (if filled in properly, of course) and be simple enough not to discourage the investigator. This is a difficult task. Much information is currently being stored on computers. Since computers can help analyze more data per unit time than scientists and statisticians, it should be routine, whenever feasible, to program all appropriate case report forms including those of Phase I.

Also, since these are times where numbers have assumed paramount importance, it is almost mandatory to use numbers and statistics whenever possible. Unfortunately, there are few respectable journals that will consider papers that do not stress numbers; the regulatory agencies demand data with detailed statistics, as do most researchers and official committees.

Many questions are appropriate in Phase II: Is the compound active? At what dose range is activity found? How does it compare to other drugs? What advantages or disadvantages does it have? How does it compare with placebo? When does the onset of action occur? Does drug resistance occur through various mechanisms? Are there other effects? What is the mechanism of action?

Some questions, such as the onset of action, are frequently not too difficult to answer. Others, such as mechanism of action, are some-times extremely problematic and very often frustrate those involved in clinical research. The true mechanism of action of most compounds is unknown. While it is easy here to enter the field of scientific philoso-phy and discuss what the mechanism of action of a drug is and how to arrive at such a point in clinical research, this point, though valid, has little practical meaning in clinical drug development. The im-portant question is, when a drug does something that is measurable and is followed by a beneficial effect in the human, how can we at-tribute the beneficial effect to what was measured when we fully realize that the most important effect might not be detected at all? Gen-erally there are two experimental designs used to detect efficacy in Phase II, the so-called open study and the now-famous double-blind study.

OPEN STUDY   For many years the open study was the experimental design used almost exclusively. In this type of study, both the investi-gator and the volunteer know that the volunteer is receiving the ex-perimental compound for the purpose indicated by the protocol. For example, if a physician is investigating a new semisynthetic penicillin, he will tell the volunteer-patient that he would like to use this semi-synthetic penicillin to treat the patient's tonsillitis.

The open study is simple and straightforward, but it has one great disadvantage, namely, in most biological systems and disease states the manifestations of a condition vary over a period of time. Anxious persons do not continue to become anxious—simply because a human being cannot stand an infinity of anxiety. A homeostatic mechanism must arise and reverse this trend for man to survive. Thus the vari-ability in human response is the first lesson of clinical research.

The variability of biological systems can frequently make the experimental design of the open study inadequate. For example, in the area of psychotherapeutics, the clinical condition can vary mark-edly. Improvement could easily be attributed to a drug when, in fact, it was part of the variation of a disease state in the untreated population that may range from 20% to 100%, because the disease state is cyclic and improves in a certain time span. It is also possible that the investi-gational new drug might be inactive. But it also follows that if given to the right population at the right time, it might be considered either 20% or 100% effective. In fact, this has been the history of many compounds in clinical drug development where claims are supposedly substantiated by studies that are not adequately designed to answer the questions asked because the studies completely ignored the natural history of the disease.

An open study is indicated when the effect of a compound will be so evident that it will not be obscured by the variability of the parameter that is to be measured, or when moral conditions prohibit the use of a placebo. Some extreme conditions in which an open study with a compound is usually done include ventricular fibrillation, terminal carcinoma, and bacteremic septicemia. Under these conditions, the use of a placebo is immoral; also, the effect of the compound will be obvious—one way or the other.

Most inadequate clinical research that has generated false claims for a compound has resulted from an open-study experimental design. Because of this, the double-blind study has come into vogue. But the open study has been overly criticized, and in its defense a few facts are in order.

The failure of the open studies occurred during the early days of clinical research. Physicians were not sufficiently trained to be objective in drug evaluation, which naturally led to false claims, both positive and negative. However, how valid would the open study be in comparison to the double-blind technique if the same investigators used it during the same period? Of course, we cannot know. It is an unfortunate state of affairs, though, if a drug is given to ten chronic, apathetic, withdrawn schizophrenics and if half of these patients begin to demonstrate an interest in their environment, that some believe this new interest could be attributed to the unsophisticated nature of the open-study, i.e., placebo effect. What these critics fail to realize is that five such schizophrenics simply do not come out of their world and approach reality because of chance or a placebo effect.

While the open study has definite limitations, it can still be of immense value, and it must not be discouraged by the scrupulous purist. Actually, an overwhelming number of dramatic drug discoveries were made by using the open technique and practically none by the double-blind method!

DOUBLE-BLIND STUDY   In a double-blind study, the investigational compound is compared either to placebo or to another compound, usually an accepted marketed drug with proven activity in the particular area being investigated. Neither the investigator nor the volunteer knows whether the volunteer is receiving the investigational new drug, placebo, or comparative drug.

With this technique, capsules or tablets should be identical in appearance, odor, and taste so that neither the investigator nor the patient can identify the substance.* While tablets may appear identical, the investgator should not overlook the possibility that there may be slight changes in odor and taste between the placebo and the investigational drug. To detect any differences he should place the tablet on his tongue. Slight changes in odor and taste can occur with some drugs if they are bottled for a sufficient period of time, particularly at room temperature. Many investigators have had experience with clever volunteers who can detect the differences in placebo or investigational drug by some qualitative difference, such as a minor discoloration or difference in taste. This occurs more frequently with tablets than with capsules, since a drug in capsule form cannot be tasted and is not visible.

A detectable qualitative difference in the tablets or capsules can reduce to equivocation an otherwise sophisticated study in a double-blind crossover test. In this type of test the investigational drug may be given to one group for a period of time and be followed without interruption by the administration of either placebo or another drug, while the opposite procedure is carried out in another group. If the volunteer thinks that what he is currently taking is different from what he took last week, his psychologic response may be radically different. This is particularly true in the field of psychotherapeutics, where placebo response is considered to be high and differences in behavior difficult to measure.

Bias or insufficient objectivity on the behalf of the investigator can also be a critical problem in therapeutic trials. If the investigator knows what the volunteer is actually taking, the experimental drug or placebo, he might not be objective in arriving at the findings of the study.

Nowadays the double-blind trial is widely accepted. One reason is that this technique appears to eliminate the possibility of error of

* Double-blind studies can also be done with parenteral dosage forms.

70

the sort involved in open studies. Indeed, it is a great relief to many to turn to the results of the double-blind trial. Despite the many assumptions inherent in this technique, it is generally accepted that if significant differences occur during a double-blind study then the difference are real, but if no differences are detected then the investigational drug is no better than placebo or the comparative drug.

Disturbingly little criticism of this design has taken place. Though it is difficult to be an ardent critic of the double-blind technique, there is a gut feeling among many distinguished clinical investigators that overreliance on this technique may result in the loss of important information. It was previously mentioned that in some areas of psychiatry the placebo response is great. The anxious or depressed patient is known as a notorious placebo responder.* Therefore, when approaching a study that compares placebo and drug, the clinical psychiatrist must consider many variables.

For example, the investigator will know there are insufficient data comparing the use of placebo versus psychotherapy or no therapy at all in this condition. Thus, he really has no true feel of what a placebo does in the depressed patient. He also knows that morally he cannot permit a depressed patient to go untreated for too long because of suicidal tendencies. Furthermore, in Phase I studies the dose that is determined for use in Phase II has certain adverse effects; therefore, he may be able to detect a difference in this manner. He knows that adverse effects reported with a placebo are frequently high, and he believes that since the placebo response is so high in depressed patients the drug must be highly effective if he detects a difference. The investigator will probably try to guess which volunteer is on a placebo and which is on the investigational drug. If he does so, he will view each subsequent clinical evaluation as a "probable drug taker" or a "probable placebo taker." On the other hand, he may do the opposite and tend to quantitate all response within a certain range on the theory that placebo is just as good as a drug in the treatment of depression.

Other problems are also involved in the double-blind technique. Double-blind trials are sometimes fixed-dose studies (though they need

* There are many who believe that the placebo response is overrated because there are few data that compare the effect of placebo with no treatment at all. There are data that demonstrate that patients who have received no treatment have a high occurrence of adverse effects.

71

not be) that can eliminate the need for imagination and dose manipulation by the clinical investigator. If the maximum tolerated dose is used, then it may be unwise to raise the dose during the study. However, this may be less of a problem than it would appear, since patients often can tolerate a significantly higher dose of some drugs than can the healthy volunteers in whom the so-called maximum tolerated dose was determined. If a dose lower than the maximum tolerated is being studied, the fixed-dose aspect of the double-blind technique can certainly be sacrificed and the dose raised if no effect is seen in the patients over a certain period of time.

During many supposedly "safe dose" studies, subtle adverse effects do occur that indicate to the investigator what volunteers are in the drug-treated population. Patients may say that they "feel funny" or "can't seem to get going." While these are extremely subjective complaints, they are real. If these occur in a significant number of volunteers and if they are drug related, then the experiment is already biased. In this situation, the investigator knows that the volunteer is taking the drug and the value of the double-blind technique is greatly diminished.

Ardent critics of the double-blind technique have produced data that raise other disturbing questions. For example, in some double-blind studies many well-established antipsychotic drugs have been found to be no better than placebo, as is illustrated in Table 10. This is particularly disturbing since the placebo response in psychotic patients is not considered to be too great. But, after careful analysis, the reasons for this phenomenom become apparent.

In most of the studies in which placebo response was equal to the antipsychotic drug, poor methodology was involved. There are many reasons for a falsely negative study, among them inadequate types or numbers of patients and sloppy observation. A single incident such as the use of an inadequate dose can create much equivocation. Table 11 demonstrates that chlorpromazine was clearly more effective than a placebo at higher doses than at lower doses. If sufficient doses had been used initially, then the results would have been less equivocal and much wasted effort would have been spared. This finding also reinforces the custom that, if feasible, the initial dose in Phase II should be close to the maximum tolerated dose. If insufficient activity is found at the maximum tolerated dose then a drug can be rejected in a shorter

72

Table 10/Double-blind Studies of the Efficacy of the Tranquilizing Drugs on Hospitalized Psychotic Patients

Drug		Number of Studies in Which	
		Drug Was More Effective Than Placebo	Drug Was Equal to Placebo
Generic Name	Trade Name		
Chlorpromazine	Thorazine Largactil	50	11
Reserpine	Serpasil	20	9
Triflupromazine	Vesprin Vespral	8	1
Perphenazine	Trilafon Fentazin	5	0
Prochlorperazine	Compazine Stemetil	7	2
Trifluoperazine	Stelazine	16	2
Fluphenazine	Prolixin Permitil	9	0
Thioridazine	Mellaril	6	1
Mepazine	Pacatal Pecazine	2	3
Promazine	Sparine	3	4
Phenobarbital		0	3

Source: By permission from JO Cole and JM Davis, Antipsychotic drugs, in L Bellak and L Loeb (eds), *The Schizophrenic Syndrome*, New York, Grune & Stratton, Inc, 1964.

period of time. This would save much of our scant clinical expertise and manpower for more worthy endeavors.

The limitations of the human experimental condition sometimes make it difficult to demonstrate significant drug differences. Once more, the best illustration is in the area of psychotropic drugs.

No significant differences in the degree of efficacy between chlorpromazine and other major antipsychotic drugs have been demonstrated, as is illustrated in Table 12. However, many investigators feel that there are substantial differences among these drugs. From a pharmacologic point of view, it is highly improbable that these different drugs with different structures behave exactly the same way in the human model. In fact, there can be substantial differences among a group of drugs even though their mean performance is identical. That

73

Table 11/Comparison of the Therapeutic Effectiveness
of Chlorpromazine As Compared
to That of Placebo, Using Controlled Studies

	Number of Studies in Which Chlorpromazine Was		
Dose Range	More Effective Than Placebo	Slightly More Effective Than Placebo	Equal to Placebo
300 mg/day or less	10	6	9
301–400 mg/day	4	3	1
401–500 mg/day	4	0	1
501–800 mg/day	14	0	0
More than 800 mg/day	9	0	0
Totals (all doses)	41	9	11

Source: By permission from JO Cole and JM Davis, Antipsychotic drugs, in L Bellak and L Loeb (eds), *The Schizophrenic Syndrome,* New York, Grune & Stratton, Inc, 1964.

no significant difference has been demonstrated just points out the need for more sophisticated experiments—regardless of whether they are open-study or double-blind.

The lack of imagination in many clinical experiments will never be corrected by the use of the double-blind design. Logistically, it is much simpler for most investigators to do an open rather than a double-blind study; the administrative steps that are involved in the beginning of a double-blind study frequently discourage the most enthusiastic investigators. If an investigator wanted to look into the effect of a particular compound on a certain disease by employing an open study, he could procure the drug and administer it to patients within a relatively short period of time. If, however, he were to perform the same investigation utilizing the double-blind technique, it would become a major effort. The drug might have to be reformulated to conform with the placebo or comparative drug. Quality control studies, along with many other administrative steps, would have to be carried out.

The major administrative effort frequently needed in the double-blind technique emphasizes the need for versatility in the clinical evaluation of drugs. Many drug discoveries have been made by

Table 12/Comparative Effectiveness of Phenothiazine Drugs Compared to Chlorpromazine As a Standard Using Controlled Studies

| | | Number of Studies in Which | | |
| | | Drug Was More Effective Than Chlorpromazine | Drug Was Equal to Chlorpromazine | Chlorpromazine Was More Effective |
Generic Name	Trade Name			
Mepazine	Pacatal	0	0	4
Promazine	Sparine	0	2	4
Triflupromazine	Vesprin	0	10	0
Perphenazine	Trilafon	0	6	0
Prochlorperazine	Compazine	0	10	0
Trifluoperazine	Stelazine	0	8	0
Thioridazine	Mellaril	0	12	0
Fluphenazine	Prolixin	0	7	0
Acetophenazine	Tindal	0	1	0
Thiopropazate	Dartal	0	1	0
Phenobarbital		0	0	6

Source: By permission from JO Cole and JM Davis, Antipsychotic drugs, in L Bellak and L Loeb (eds), *The Schizophrenic Syndrome*, New York, Grune & Stratton, Inc, 1964.

clinicians who have witnessed an unexpected observation and then explored it with rapidity and enthusiasm. The double-blind technique would certainly discourage this process since it is essential with this design not to deviate from the protocol.

Some investigators who are involved in initial Phase II studies prefer to utilize the open study before embarking on a double-blind study in order to acquire a "feel" for the experimental compound. The investigator dealing with a new experimental compound feels—and rightly so—that he should acquire the knowledge of whether the drug is both relatively efficacious and safe. With an open study, he can manipulate the dose frequently and eventually select the optimum dose range for testing in the subsequent double-blind study. After the results of two or three open studies are evaluated, later investigators can go right to the double-blind technique.

In summary, the double-blind study is not always necessary. If ten hyperthyroid patients all become clinically euthyroid within the first week and all PBIs are within the normal range, then a placebo is not needed to prove the fact of efficacy. But as one CDD has noted, "The growing literature of scientific clinical investigation reinforces the principle: When in doubt, rule out the subjective response."* This frequently means the use of the double-blind study.

To Determine the Margin of Safety

One of the most difficult aspects of clinical research is to determine a dose that is as efficacious as the maximum tolerated dose, yet as far from this level as practical. This is not easy, for many factors play an important role in determining the margin of safety. In this discussion, dosing and duration will be emphasized for simplicity.

If an antibiotic is 100% effective at 100 mg, then it should be evaluated at a dosage of 50 mg. If it is also 100% effective at 50 mg, then the dose should be reduced once more. Multiple doses can be studied simultaneously if it is feasible and if there is no great risk to the patient. If this same antibiotic is 100% effective at 100 mg for a period of ten days, it could be tested for a period of five days at the same dose or lower.

Under certain conditions, steroids can be equally efficacious if given every other day instead of daily, which, hopefully, would reduce the incidence of adverse effects. If, however, this might reduce the therapeutic effect, the dose should not be lowered.

Many times it is not known whether it is the peak concentration of a drug in the plasma, its duration, or a combination of both that is responsible for a drug effect. By adjusting doses to accentuate either the dose or the duration it may be possible to dissociate an efficacious effect from the adverse effect. Thus by *raising* the dose and *decreasing* the duration of administration, the incidence of adverse effects may be dramatically reduced with little impact on efficacy. The rule, therefore, is to adjust the dose and the duration of dosing in order to increase safety without sacrificing the desired objectives of the drug.

The major problem in most clinical circumstances results from dealing with humans in a biological screen. Multiple colonies of hu-

* Sheldon G Gilgore (speech given at the Symposium on Progress in Drug Research, sponsored by the Pharmaceutical Manufacturing Association, in Washington, D.C., March 6, 1969).

man volunteers cannot be recruited very easily, but even if this were possible, the cost of doing so would be prohibitive. If only the acute administration of a compound is being studied, as is sometimes done with a hypoglycemic agent, then the titration of the dose is rather important before the drug can be made available to the general population. On the other hand, if a compound is being studied for its antidepressant activity, titration is not so important since it is difficult to assess the dose range where sufficient antidepressant activity occurs, and even more arduous to show a meaningful difference in response between two groups on different dose levels. Under these circumstances, one should administer a sufficient amount of drug, while avoiding a prohibitive adverse effect profile.

Many claim that not enough emphasis has been placed on the development of a definable margin of safety. However, those who choose to pursue this objective to its extremes are not aware of the limitations of clinical research. All responsible investigators should seek to define the margin of safety within reason and constantly review the data, particularly in reference to the dose-duration relationship. But the value of the golden mean should not be ignored.

Phase II studies usually last from a few days to months and sometimes longer. Tentative conclusions about a drug can be radically changed in Phase III because of new findings. The optimum time to evaluate the margin of safety in a definitive manner is after Phase III studies have been completed. Only then can one decide whether the increased incidence of headache due to the investigational drug is a reasonable price to be paid for the beneficial effects accrued. Only then can a "me too" sulfonylurea be judged inadequate for the general population because of a 25% incidence of severe headaches. Only then can an antitumor compound be joyously accepted because there is only a 25% incidence of severe headache in the drug-treated group.

Unfortunately, the judgment of a reasonable margin of safety is sometimes a function of temperament rather than fact.

Serendipity

Serendipity—the gift of making fortunate chance discoveries—has a special meaning in the pharmaceutical world. There are numerous examples of this phenomenon that have played an important part in drug discovery. A classic example is the use of DDS (Dapsone) against malaria. DDS is used in the treatment of leprosy; by chance it was discovered that patients with this disease who had taken DDS over a long period of time had a low incidence of malaria. The cause and effect relationship of this observation has now been substantiated by time.

Many investigators have, at one time or another, sought to plan on the occurrence of serendipity in the clinical setting. But serendipity is a capricious goddess, and to plan for serendipity is, in all truth, a contradiction of the term.

To maximize the chances of finding an unexpected effect of the compound, one should simply increase the number of laboratory screens in any clinical study. Thus, more parameters are measured and the chance of discovering an unexpected effect is increased. Another way is to test the drug against more than one condition. For example, the medicinal chemist might look at the potential hypoglycemic candidate and wonder how the drug will be metabolized. If he thinks that it is metabolized similarly to folic acid, he would speculate on the compound's activity against carcinoma or other conditions where antifols have proven activity.

The number of laboratory tests performed with compounds having adverse effects that are not considered a severe problem (e.g., progestins or estrogens) is usually less than the number done with an unknown structure or with compounds that have significant target-organ toxicity in animals. If a clinical investigator ordered six liver-function tests instead of the normal two or three with the estrogen or progesterone analogue, he might discover an important unexpected effect. While there are many investigators who like to evaluate the animal data and then select what tests should be done in man, it is becoming more common to do a fixed battery of many tests regardless of the nature of the drug.

The argument that too many tests will produce confusing data falls flat. The only real danger is that too many laboratory studies may produce a red herring, an abnormal laboratory value that is not a drug effect but an error in laboratory technique. This red herring could upset the regulatory agencies, e.g., the FDA, and result in an inordinate amount of increased work and delays in order to show that the effect was not drug related. Those involved in clinical drug development know how frustrating this experience can be.

Phase III

The intellectual challenge and the excitement of anticipation surrounding the initial trials in man occur during Phase I and Phase II studies; the challenge of Phase III does not compare to the drama of the transition from animal to man. The emergence of this viewpoint is probably related to semantic difficulties. If the objective of clinical research was described as the effort to bring to the general population drugs that are beneficial and safe, then Phase III clearly is as important as Phases I and II. It is interesting, however, that the medical departments in some pharmaceutical companies have divided their clinical research manpower into Phase I and II sections to accommodate the different types of expertise needed.

In Phase III studies, the experimental drug is given to a large group of people (usually a few hundred to a thousand, occasionally many more) to determine

1. Whether the drug will continue to perform as expected from Phase I and II studies

2. Whether unexpected events, such as new types of efficacy or adverse effects not previously detected, will occur

3. Whether there is an interaction with other drugs that are taken by the population

In Phase III studies, genetic differences, both familial and ethnic, may be detected. For example, if primaquine were screened in 300 Caucasians in Phases I and II, its hemolytic effect in Negroes could probably pass unnoticed until Phase III studies were instituted. Chronic drug effects, such as eye changes that occur with long-term administration of phenothiazines, can only be detected during Phase III. These are only a few of the examples that one could cite to illustrate the various events that might be discovered in large-scale studies.

If a drug causes an undesired effect in less than 1% of the population, then the adverse effect falls within the third standard deviation of the normal distribution curve and thus is unlikely to be detected in small populations. The purpose of Phase III studies is to search, in a large population, for certain characteristics of a drug on the normal distribution curve.

Phase III is a rather large challenge. It is much more than an attempt to confirm the findings of Phases I and II. It is an attempt at total identification of the drug. But what is not always appreciated or realized in Phase III studies is the amount of effort necessary to generate and retrieve essential information.

Phase III studies are not so well-controlled as early clinical studies because of the magnitude of the effort. The physician involved in these studies usually evaluates more patients less often. He is frequently reluctant to devote the inordinate amount of his working time necessary to fill in the case report forms consistently and completely. The investigators who are involved in Phase I and II studies are frequently full-time academic clinicians with time to wonder, but the Phase III investigator often is a practicing clinician without this luxury. The problems that he confronts are quite different and very real. If agranulocytosis occurs in one in a thousand, what is the verdict? Was it due to the experimental drug? Was it due to another drug? Was it drug related? This type of analysis becomes particularly frustrating, for many adverse effects do occur in any given group of 1,000 people due to chance alone, rather than drug-related factors.

Phase III studies lack the respectable aura they deserve, and this is to be deplored because many important drug decisions rest on the results of Phase III studies.

So-called Phase IV

The term "Phase IV" is today not so well accepted as the terms "Phase I, II, and III." Phase IV involves studies that are done after a drug has been approved by the FDA for general use. As a rule, these studies are directed by the medical departments of marketing divisions in pharmaceutical firms. Since they often are geared to advertising the drug and explaining the conditions for which it is effective, they are sometimes viewed with little esteem. But there are few who realize the great problem in getting information to the physician, particularly in our present era where many good compounds for the same diseases are being marketed without profound differences in efficacy for a particular indication.

There are indications that Phase IV research, on occasion, is becoming more imaginative than that carried on during Phases I, II, or

III. In this situation, the physician working on Phase IV studies may be involved in seeking out more meaningful information about why a physician should use a drug. Thus, while the research physician must demonstrate to the medical community and the FDA that a drug works and that it is safe, the Phase IV physicians must not only show that a drug works, but how it is different and perhaps more beneficial than other drugs with similar activity.

Nonetheless, the role of the Phase IV physician is usually a thankless one. He lacks the prestige of the research physician and he is frequently deficient in the necessary scientific expertise to mingle with the "experts" of the drug cognoscenti. Because the physician directing Phase IV studies reports to the leader of marketing and sales divisions, there is a feeling that he is less scientific and, therefore, not worthy of scientific respect.

The nature of our time demands that his role should change, and there are now some indications that this is occurring. Some say that a drug is not truly known until it has been used by the general population for at least a few years. Unexpected happenings both in the area of efficacy and adverse effects frequently occur while the drug is "out there." Therefore, it should be the responsibility of the Phase IV physician to monitor the drug closely and to initiate new studies that further identify the compound. He should also advise the marketing and sales divisions of the limitations of the drug's activity and guard against exaggerated promotions. Whereas these are already the purported duties of the Phase IV physician, too often he has not been able to carry them out because of his limited status.

What is needed in this area are men with research competence who can appreciate the scientific aspects of the experimental compound, but who can also communicate with the marketing divisions of the industry, the academic authorities, and the government.

There are few who can fill this role today. Only when this situation is altered will the total medical expertise required by the pharmaceutical institutions be brought to fruition.

Reference

1. Duncan WAM: The importance of metabolism studies in relation to drug toxicity. Proc Europ Soc Drug Toxicity 2:67, 1963.

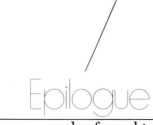

Epilogue

"The proper study of mankind is man"

ALEXANDER POPE

We have seen in the preceding chapters that a drug embarks on a long journey before it reaches the physician as part of his armamentarium. This entire process is guided by the clinical drug developer. We have seen too that the animal screen now gives us the only objective data upon which we decide if and how we shall proceed with a drug candidate into man. While there is a significant degree of predictability, both from the point of efficacy and toxicity, from the animal screen to man, there is also a significant degree of unpredictability that unfortunately prevents reasonable certitude.

The overwhelming fact is that the present preclinical evaluation of a drug is simply not a very good way of making new drug discoveries. But it is also quite evident that this condition is not going to change within the near future.

Let us examine the function of the current drug discovery system and see where and how improvements can be made.

In the area of medicinal chemistry there is much talent and a multitude of available compounds that have not been evaluated for biologic activity. Many think the chemical aspect of drug development is the most advanced in the pharmaceutical world today.

It has been said that if the biologist can tell the chemist what specifications a compound should have, the chemist will have no problem producing the required structure. The biologist's problem is that he can only request a compound that lowers cholesterol in the rat or in another species and then *hope* that it will be efficacious in hypercholesterolemic patients.

82

There is almost a pathetic irony in this type of reasoning because it is based on so many assumptions. For we have already seen that there is no reason to believe that the rat has any more predictive value than the toad or the gorilla. Similarly, why assume that a drug that lowers cholesterol in the rat will do so in the normal person, let alone in the hyperchoesterolemic patient. Even if the compound does lower cholesterol in the normal or hypercholesterolemic human, there is no proof that its activity will benefit the patient. It is quite conceivable that if the cholesterol is lowered through the wrong mechanism of action we could aggravate the complications of atherosclerosis.

Thus, while the medicinal chemist can produce a compound that is a feasible agent in lowering cholesterol, he cannot predict whether or not a compound possessing certain biologic characteristics in the animal screen will counteract the etiology of hypercholesterolemia. He must await the findings of the biologists.

The biologists who are involved in such animal studies must, by nature, be endowed with an abundance of energy and optimism. It takes a particular temperament to believe that a compound that decreases rat paw edema will be an effective anti-inflammatory drug in man or that a new plant extract that reverses reserpine-induced depression in certain animals will be an effective antidepressant in clinical practice.

The remarkable aspect of the current drug discovery system is that there are drugs that affect rat paw edema or reserpine-induced depression and actually are also effective in man. One must have the greatest respect for the brave toxicologist whose job it is to produce toxicity in animals. After having done so he frequently is not sure what will occur in man with the experimental compound, and yet he is called upon to relate the toxicological findings to the clinical picture.

After the endless hours spent in preparing a candidate for human consumption, the drug comes into the hands of the clinical pharmacologist for Phase I evaluation. But this stage may never be reached if some disturbing toxicity occurs in the animal studies. For example, if an exciting novel bronchodilator causes a peculiar deposition in the rat prostate it might never reach man for evaluation. The compound must be judged safe enough in relation to the animal data for testing.

The fate of many potential candidates can be seen by viewing the path of a hypocholesterolemic agent effective in lowering the cholesterol in both normal and hypercholesterolemic rats, dogs, and monkeys.

This level of efficacy indicates that it is a candidate for clinical trials. First, it is evaluated in approximately 20 normal volunteers at increasing doses. Significant nausea is observed in about 60% of the population, yet no hypocholesterolemic effect is observed. Then the compound is tested in, perhaps, 20 hypercholesterolemic patients at the maximum tolerated dose, and again no lipid lowering is observed. The compound, for all practical purposes, is dead as a clinical candidate and most of the effort expended by the scientific team has been fruitless.

Occasionally, and despite the high cost, a second candidate in the series is chosen for evaluation, but once more no activity is observed. The cost and manpower then involved in testing the third and fourth candidates are frequently prohibitive; as a result, the exciting new structural series is abandoned.

If, by good fortune, the initial compound has shown some activity, then other candidates in the chemical series may be evaluated. The theory behind this is that there is a higher probability that a useful clinical candidate will be developed. Unfortunately, these efforts often fail and the clinical pharmacologists must then retract their enthusiasm as the preclinical scientists retreat once again into the world of medicinal chemistry and animal studies.

The uncertainty of this approach illustrates some basic problems in our present system of drug development. Also, much of the time, effort, and expense expended in our present system often is lost.

A more certain approach would be to evaluate many hypocholesterolemic agents in man after minimal animal pharmacology and toxicology studies, since the most active drug in the animal will not necessarily produce parallel activity in man. By increasing the number of drugs evaluated in man, a better understanding of the animal screens can be obtained and a more precise animal-man correlation can be made. Why was the least and not the most active drug in the rat screen much more efficacious in man? The pharmacologist would attempt to answer this question by doing more studies and then altering his screening techniques. In so doing he aids the medicinal chemist in planning his strategy for synthesizing chemicals that have relevance to man.

Let me emphasize that most new drugs can be evaluated safely in man with only a minimal amount of animal data. If, after the initial test for activity in man, the new compound is discovered to have potential, *then* extensive pharmacology and toxicology should be done before extensive clinical trials are initiated. Unfortunately, this reasoning is not widely accepted today.

In any logical system, a rigid policy of clinical drug development that relies heavily on preclinical testing would be considered irrational. It makes little sense to study drugs in areas that are predominantly peripheral to the basic problem. It makes even less sense to follow this arduous procedure when a suitable short cut in the form of clinical trials is available.

Since man is the primary point of interest in the development of new drugs, it is man who should be studied. The medicinal chemists can produce new compounds and the biologists can evaluate the initial activity of these compounds, but we cannot *discover* the potential of many new compounds until they are studied in man.

Applied and Pioneering Research

In the area of any research endeavor, there are two major categories that deserve emphasis: Applied research and pioneering research.

Applied research can be defined as the constant application of known principles in an unspectacular way. It usually is basically unimaginative but extremely necessary, since it is the background of all research organizations.

Pioneering research can be defined as that type of endeavor in which something most unusual and challenging is discovered. An immediate pragmatic use does not necessarily follow this type of research.

An immunologic quantitatitve method to measure circulating insulin levels is a recent example of pioneering research in medicine. This method was a spectacular breakthrough in the area of diabetic research. Immediately following this discovery, the applied researchers used this new method to study the insulin levels in diabetes, fasting states, acromegaly, hypothyroidism, and Cushing's disease. The pioneers will now read and evaluate the data generated by the applied researchers of diabetes. And when another dramatic breakthrough occurs, the applied researchers will begin work anew to give additional fuel to the pioneering mind.

These two types of research, the combination of both applied and pioneering, spell discovery, and can provide the logical answer for successful drug discovery today, particularly by large organizations such as exist in the pharmaceutical industry.

With the present climate of opinion, the emphasis in clinical investigations is on applied research, and pioneering research has been largely ignored. The primary reason is that Food and Drug Administration regulations now require that a vast amount of applied research be carried out in order to demonstrate the effectiveness of a new drug. Unfortunately, this demand for increased applied research comes at a time when there is an increased scientific demand for new knowledge. Yet the amount of time and manpower required to carry out the applied research tasks has served to eclipse most attempts at pioneering research.

The clinical development of a new hypocholesterolemic drug requires a very large amount of applied research efforts. Perhaps 20 double-blind studies, along with many open long-term studies, are needed to demonstrate whether the drug is efficacious and safe enough to approve for general use. The laborious effort is extremely necessary, but does not lend itself to producing imaginative or productive new knowledge. Yet it strains the available manpower in this field and leaves little time or few experts to carry out the more imaginative work that is essential in a discovery system.

Given the time and available manpower, a pioneering approach to the study of a new hypocholesterolemic agent might be an attempt to place a minicamera on the tip of a cardiac catheter. One could then attempt to photograph the atheromatous coronary plaques of a small population. This population would be divided into two groups—one given the experimental drug and the other placebo. After awhile one could then rephotograph the coronaries. Only then would there be an answer to the critical question: Does this hypocholesterolemic drug decrease or prevent the increase of the size of the fatal coronary plaque? It is unfortunate that pioneering research attempts such as this and others are not more common, particularly since it is highly probable that without pioneering research, drug discovery will be unnecessarily delayed.

Why aren't more drugs evaluated in man? Why isn't pioneering research a more integral part of our drug development system since the rationale supporting these positions is basically sound? The answers to these questions would fill a volume, but a few broad observations may shed some light on the puzzle.

The era of support and interest in medical research appears to have diminished, and a concerned citizenry is now focusing its attention on social problems. In such times it can be unwise to call for an increase in human experimentation with drugs. While society is willing to accept the hazards of the space program, this is not the case with drugs. We have seen that drugs have tremendous social overtones. For example, even if the FDA believed there was no evidence that cyclamates cause tumors in people and were, therefore, safe for consumption, it could scarcely hold to this position when confronted by the mass media and the Senate hearings. How can the commissioner of the FDA be required to use scientific judgment and at the same time be constantly called before Congress and scrutinized by those who may have no great scientific knowledge but do possess the ability to communicate to large numbers of people?

These factors make it difficult for the FDA to rule objectively unless it somehow establishes a scientific expertise that is free and independent of its regulatory function. Under such an arrangement, if a judgment is made that X drug is acceptably safe, and, subsequently, it is shown to cause cataracts in small numbers of people, the commissioner of the FDA would not be unfairly criticized. If this scientific body is considered highly capable, it will not be assailed for having made a judgment that could not possibly have foreseen the occurrence of cataracts. Whether this scientific body should be part of or separate from the FDA needs careful thought.

The FDA's sensitive position naturally influences the academic and pharmaceutical communities since it regulates a substantial portion of clinical research carried on by these groups. Even if there were a desire to increase the quantity and quality of clinical investigation it would be difficult. The FDA must keep a watchful eye on studies that are unusual or that employ larger than ordinary doses.

Thus we have a subliminal vicious circle wherein the FDA requests that studies be as safe as possible and the academic and pharmaceutical industry conducts safe-as-possible studies. The ultimate effect of this process would be that no one is accountable for the occasional and sometimes unavoidable drug tragedy.

Beyond this preoccupation with safety is the reality that there is no identifiable movement in the drug community to pave the way for increased clinical research. This further compounds the vicious circle, and the final result is a relatively unproductive drug discovery system.

How then will the importance of increased marginal and pioneering clinical research ever become an accepted reality? "Certitude is for fools," said the Scottish skeptic David Hume, and yet I suspect that the distinguished philosopher was referring to absolute certitude. There is a thing, however, called "reasonable certitude," to which wise men, not fools, ascribe. It is a thing that says it is obvious that certain things must be done before a general solution to any problem is effected. Is there a solution to drug dilemmas that can be proposed with reasonable certitude? Hume was a skeptic, but he was by no means a cynic.

I believe that there is, indeed, a possible solution. The first step is to understand the nature of the problem. This means that those significant individuals in the academic, pharmaceutical, and government communities must understand the nature of clinical drug development and the principles upon which it is based. This step is critical. There is a profound ignorance of this area and much of the opinion generated is therefore erroneous. Who can tell what academicians will say once given the privilege of seeing the total picture? It will be interesting to observe. The same can be said of the men in government and even the pharmaceutical community.

How can this come to be? How can different people in different fields, who have never been trained in clinical drug development, ever come to know this obscure medical specialty?

I should like to propose that the major pharmaceutical firms make available for learning purposes the facts about how some of their prototype drugs were developed. Then the evaluation of the course of a drug from the test tube to the shelf of the pharmacist will finally be open to examination and criticism. Hopefully, a meaningful dialogue can then ensue. It is also imperative that a system or residency be established to train the much-needed clinical drug developers.

In addition, there must be an alternative movement to increase the quality and quantity of applied and pioneering clinical research. This will be extremely difficult to accomplish unless there is strong societal support. Although history is not an exact science and is subjected to various interpretations, some facts do stand out clearly. The initiation of the Kefauver hearings delivered a significant blow to our drug discovery system (Fig. 8). The regulations that shortly followed merely sealed this blow in the pages of history. Strangely enough, this phenomenon is largely ignored and does not receive the attention it deserves. The message is not difficult to decipher.

The hearings initially focused on the cost of drugs. Public response began to pale, and within a short period of time the emphasis changed to the subject of adverse effects of drugs. The bad aspects of drugs are attractive subjects to the public and the media, and the hearings, therefore, became very popular. During this time the thalidomide event occurred and dramatically hastened the passage of the regulations. Thalidomide, therefore, exemplified the spirit of the regulations, and understandably the key issue was and remains that of safety for the consumer. The FDA is the official consumer representative responding to those forces which demand the elimination of risk. Many critics of the FDA do not take this into consideration and unjustly accuse it of making arbitrary decisions.

The Kefauver hearings plus the tremendous force of consumerism generated in the decade of the 1960s have forced the FDA into an extreme position of *primum non nocere* ("above all do no harm") instead of the more positive one of "first do some good for the patient." Since the society has mandated this (at least apparently so), then the FDA must comply, for that is its function. This augurs poorly for drug discovery. We must realize that most diseases are still with us and are not, contrary to what one reads or hears, about to be cured. The elimination of the great diseases of the cardiovascular, nervous, metabolic, and other systems looms far on the horizon of time. The current movement to remove the FDA from the jurisdiction of HEW and place it into a larger, nonscientific consumer agency would expose our drug discovery system to even greater consumer pressures leading inevitably to a further decrease in new drugs.

Unfortunately, the problem of increasing the productivity of clinical research cannot be solved by a reorganization of the FDA, for the very nature of this organization precludes it from taking any kind of risk—theoretical or actual. Yet risk is an essential part of drug discovery.

It appears, therefore, that the next logical step is to decentralize Phases I and II from direct FDA control. Regional peer groups either

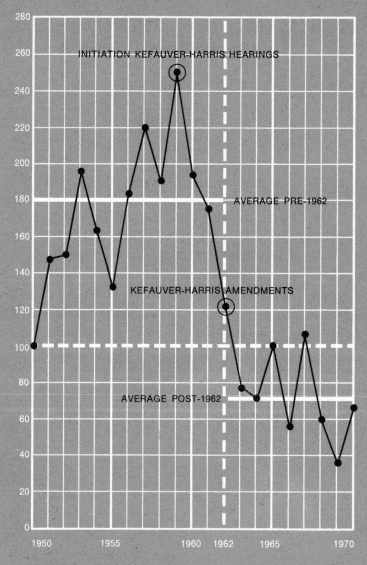

Figure 8 / New single chemical-entity introductions since 1950. (From P de Haen, *Nonproprietary Name Index,* New York, Paul de Haen, Inc, 1971. Redrawn from illustration by JP Curran.)

in medical schools or in medical centers would review research protocols submitted by the investigator and monitor the studies. Thus the critical aspect of clinical research would be brought under the guidance of scientific experts (the FDA is primarily a regulatory agency, not a scientific one), and the FDA would be relieved from many unnecessary pressures. If, after the initial studies, the experimental compound is judged to be "marketable," then it should rightly fall under the direct supervision of the FDA. The FDA commissioner and his staff then can have the benefit of reviewing "peered data," which can be most helpful in decision-making. From that point, additional scientific muscle power should be made available to the FDA to advise and review the clinical program designed to bring the new drug to the armamentarium of the physician.

However, even if the above were to come about, one great obstacle would still remain—that of legal retribution. It is no secret that clinical investigators are running scared and will perform only those studies in which the risk is minimal. This surely is an unhealthy trend, and even decentralization would not be of much help. The regional peer group would come under direct social pressure and be afraid to err, for there would be no legal forgiveness. The Congress must pass some form of no-fault legislation for the peer group and the clinical investigators. The issue is a critical one, for without its resolution no reorganization of the FDA or any other proposal can succeed. The courts have an unhealthy handle on the science of clinical research, and this issue must be resolved soon.

There are indeed legitimate pros and cons for the aforementioned proposals. Nevertheless the options are few, and something reasonable must be done—soon. The academic, pharmaceutical, and relevant government bodies must all participate in structuring this new endeavor. For only then will false idols topple, reason emerge, and clinical research be given its proper value and due respect.

If this does not occur, I have a great pessimism that our society will fail to deliver critical drugs to its present constituents.

Appendix

This appendix contains a very brief review of the current FDA regulations that are required to evaluate a new drug in man on a limited basis and, eventually, in the general population.

Investigational New Drugs are medicinal compounds with a proposed indication, dosage, or dosage form that has not been approved by the FDA. In such cases, an exemption permitting their investigational use in humans is required for Phase I, II, or III studies. The exemption is in a form entitled "A Notice of Claimed Investigational Exemption for a New Drug" (IND Form FD-1571).

Drugs that are already approved by the FDA require no IND to permit a clinical study (usually of the so-called Phase IV variety) that involves an indication, dosage, or dosage form approved in the package insert.

The IND filed with the FDA contains information to support the manufacturer's claim that the drug can be safely administered to man under specified conditions. It includes, among other things, information pertaining to (1) the animal toxicology and pharmacology of the drug, (2) a qualitative and quantitative description of the dosage forms and details of proposed production techniques and analytical assay, (3) the design, or protocol, of the study, (4) a form 1572 (for Phase I and II studies) or 1573 (for Phase III) signed by each investigator to confirm his understanding of the drug under study and his responsibilities relevant to FDA regulations, and (5) an agreement by the sponsor to monitor the study and report findings to the FDA at specified periods of time.

Under current FDA regulations, Phase I studies can begin 30 days after the IND is submitted to the FDA, provided that FDA does not comment adversely on the intentions of the research and the design of the study. Following completion of Phase I studies, a submission of the results is made to the FDA, whereupon Phase II and III studies may be initiated, usually without awaiting official response or comment.

In Phase I and II studies, written consent by volunteers is required. In Phase III studies, written consent is not required, but verbal consent is necessary and should be verifiable.

After Phase III studies have shown that the drug is safe and efficacious under the conditions of use prescribed in the proposed labeling, the sponsor can then submit a New Drug Application (NDA) to the FDA for its approval. The NDA is a document intended to demonstrate that the clinical data are sufficient to justify that the drug is safe and efficacious for the recommended indications. It is a highly complex form, frequently running 20 or 30 volumes and thousands of pages, that contains almost every item of information concerning the new drug and related drugs, but particularly data from clinical studies.* While the FDA is legally required to review this form within 180 days, it can, for various reasons, label the NDA as incomplete, whereupon the 180-day clock begins to run anew, or may choose to state that it has not been filed because of gross deficiencies in the submission.

After the NDA is approved and the drug made available to the physician, the manufacturer is required to submit to the FDA new information relating to animal and human findings, along with production and assay methods not previously submitted or not previously known. This must be done every three months during the first year, every six months during the second, and annually thereafter. If an unexpected adverse effect is attributed to the drug, it must be reported to the FDA within 15 days.

This review of the administrative steps that are required to take a new drug from animal to man would seem to indicate that it is a rather simple and straightforward procedure, but it is not. There are a multitude of factors that enter into the approval of an NDA; this results in a complicated and laborious procedure which usually requires continuous interaction between the manufacturer and the FDA.

* A recent NDA contained over 72,000 pages in 167 volumes, and these in triplicate. In Great Britain approximately 860 pages are required in an application; in Switzerland, 160 pages.

58469